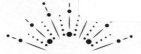

MODERN

MAGIC

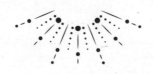

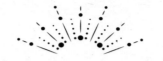

MODERN MAGIC

Stories,

Rituals, and

Spells for

Contemporary

Witches

Michelle Tea

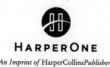

HarperOne

An Imprint of HarperCollins*Publishers*

HarperCollins books may be purchased for educational, business, or sales promotional use. For information, please email the Special Markets Department at SPsales@harpercollins.com.

FIRST EDITION

Designed by Bonni Leon-Berman

Library of Congress Cataloging-in-Publication Data has been applied for.

ISBN 978-0-06-337819-3

24 25 26 27 CPI 10 9 8 7 6 5 4 3 2

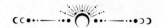

For

Phyllis Mansfield,

grandmother &

latent witch

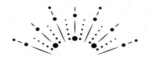

CONTENTS

Introduction 1

1. Welcome to My Coven	21
2. Patron Saints and Other Witches	35
3. Luck, Good and Bad	53
4. Divine!	69
5. Kitchen Witchery and Mystical Snacktivism	91
6. Familiarize Yourself	105
7. Catch Your Breath	119
8. Hex Marks the Spot	137
9. Interlude: What Are We Even Doing?	155
10. Dreaming Is Free	173
11. House Work	185
12. Witch Panic	205
13. Bring Me Love, and Sex. And Love.	229

Appendix: Modern Magic Book List/My Bookshelves 243

Acknowledgments 245

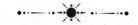

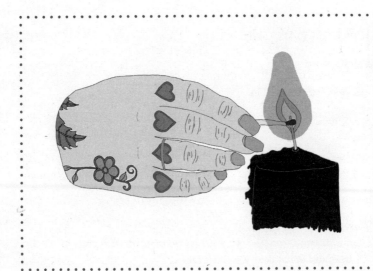

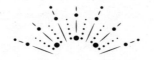

INTRODUCTION

I was a teen witch. It was the '80s, it was New England, I was goth—the scene was set. The first time I stepped into an occult store, I thought, *yes*. The weird, herbal smells, the employees similarly clad in black, the jars containing strange tufts of dried flowers, the candles. The candles! I've always been partial to candles. I felt that, with my abiding interest in the supernatural, my childhood hobby of mixing every liquid in the house and calling it "potion"—not to mention the influence of all the low-key spooky women in my life, mom and Nana and aunts who liked to get wired on cups of Tetley tea, chain-smoke, and talk about their weird dreams or reincarnation—well, I felt like I was always a witch. It just took a bit of cultural bullying and the discovery of an occult store to bring me home.

Later, when I was in my early twenties transitioning out of the goth subculture I'd huddled in through my teens, trading in some of my widow's weeds for clothing that incorporated *color*, I thought about what I was morphing out of, who I would continue to become. What did I want to bring with me? I wondered how magic would remain a part of my life as I moved away from emo music and aesthetics and into the worlds and concepts that newly compelled me—feminism, activism, queerness. A burgeoning understanding of myself as working class, with all the politics and psychologies that lens offered. Amazingly, witchcraft didn't feel less relevant but, rather, increasingly relevant as I explored these new areas of life.

As right as the witch label felt, however, I've often wondered if I am putting on airs. I mean, I don't own a robe (a cape, yes, wool, gorgeous, timeless); I've never been initiated into a coven (despite lots of tight friendships with cool, eerie weirdos); I can't really say if what I'm doing in front of my altar with my candles is "Wiccan," or "pagan," or what! I let full moon after full moon go dark in the sky without ever putting my crystals out for charging. And yet I find, again and again, that I want—I need—to have a regular practice of communicating with the Universe, with everything I can't see but *feel* is there. I need to see my intentions in the form of a waxy candle growing hotter. I need to scent my room with smoke and feel the otherworldly residue of it in my hair. I like paging through books of spells and selecting one that could help me snag my desire; I like the connection it gives to the past. I like brainstorming my own weird spells using "magical tools" I grab from a craft store or Target, my kitchen, or my kid's toy box. Is this witchcraft?

Over the years—and it's been some years, decades!—I've increasingly settled into myself as a witch. I've come to understand it's not an elite club, no one is going to call me a "poser" for not properly celebrating Yule or neglecting to make a jar of full moon water. The gorgeousness of a modern magic tradition is that we get to curate it to suit us exactly. We can select

INTRODUCTION

traditions and practices from the past, from our own ancestry and heritage; we get to glean spiritual inspiration from the internet or from our friends. We can practice when we are moved and inspired and we can put it down for a sec if we're not feeling it. We can worship and feel devotional to mythical beings that resonate, or we can make an offering to our own highest self. *Modern Magic* has no rules, is proudly magpie, while keeping an eye out for cultural appropriation, as we have learned the lessons of the New Age hodgepodge that came before us. We can do the work to learn if a spiritual practice is "open"—meaning, the culture it belongs to has generously offered, or made peace with, sharing it with the larger world—versus "closed" practices, those rituals that are reserved for the folks who are truly a part of the originating culture. For the white people among us, unlearning racism and white supremacy must be part of our spiritual practice; respecting that there are traditions that are not for us is an important aspect of that work. Approaching traditions outside your own with appreciation and respectful curiosity—versus a white supremacist belief that everything is theirs for the taking—makes a difference. (Also, a stance of appreciation and respectful curiosity in general just might be a spiritual practice in its own right!)

Witchcraft has always been feminist. Witches—women—were the first doctors, the ones who knew herbs and plants could help and heal a body, the ones who understood the mysteries of birth, who helped demystify it for new mothers in their roles as midwives. Barbara Ehrenreich and Deirdre English spoke of these wise women in their seminal feminist pamphlet, *Witches,*

Midwives & Nurses: A History of Women Healers, saying, "her magic was the science of her time." The Royal College of Nursing in Scotland is currently funding a massive research project to find evidence of practicing midwives among the 4,000 individuals accused of witchcraft in Scotland between 1563 and 1736 (over 80 percent female, of course). There is a movement to absolve these "witches" of antiquity of witchcraft, and reclaim them as nurses, or simply as independent women who went against the grain of their times. But there is *also* a movement among contemporary witches to recognize them as our foremothers, reclaiming the pejorative *witch* as not only the accurate term for a person whose spiritual practice deals with the manipulation of energy, belief in the power of nature, and embrace of female deities, but also as a powerful cultural term for women, through the ages, who refused to be controlled, to dim their personal power or disavow their connection to the great unknown.

As a young feminist, I was thrilled to see that the magical practice I'd begun dabbling in during high school actually supported my empowerment and independence as a woman. In the *maiden, mother, crone* triad of femme life-stages that many pagan traditions honor, I saw for the first time the phases of a female's life, from youth through old age, held with respect and honor. Maidens weren't young and dumb, ditzy and foolish; they held the wisdom of wild mind, the innocence and insight of a beginner. Mothers weren't barefoot and pregnant, boring, or self-sacrificing; they didn't even have to be *mothers* per se. They were simply women at a moment when their physical power and the power of their lived experience synced up, allowing their dynamic creative energy to be sunk into any sphere at all—motherhood, sure, but also the pursuit of art or thought, sex, business, or relationships.

But it was probably the revered archetype of the crone that most moved me, at that moment in my youth. I'd seen the maiden and mother celebrated, if perversely, in the larger culture, but never had I seen a femme at the end of her life honored and revered for all that she'd survived, for the accumulation of her knowledge, for the way her body bowed to the forces of nature, having squeezed every drop of life from her precious muscle, bone, and flesh. Never had I seen an elderly woman's proximity to death approached with awe and curiosity. The crone in mass culture was a dithering fool, the other side of the ditzy girl coin: a little gross, a little scary, but mostly sad and powerless. With witchcraft, I caught a vision of the crone as uniquely powerful, still sexual, even, still a cultural force in her community—still *alive*, a goddess, dammit. Within witchcraft, women and femmes got to take up unapologetic space during all phases of life, and this revelation was one of deep relief to me then, at the tender age of twenty. While my own life was still largely unimaginable, witchcraft and feminism gave me a shadowy sense of how I might make the most of my time on this Earth, and be emboldened to chase down the experiences that called to me.

The empowerment that witchcraft offers is not unique to those who identify as women, and it has become only more attractive as traditionally marginalized people take up an increasing amount of space in our culture. The demise of organized, patriarchal religions has been making headlines for years now, as has the story running alongside it—as people leave churches in droves, they come with curiosity to practices that have long been demonized or ridiculed by patriarchal religions. Queer people of all genders find uncompromising acceptance and celebration for their sacred queerness within witchcraft. Indeed, it was effeminate men, men who defied the gender roles of their times, who were cruelly used as kindling—"faggots"—to burn the femme witches of the Middle Ages in Europe. Powerful women who disobey the orders to be meek and ignorant have always shared outlaw status with men who withstood the pressure to be cruel or hard or not love one another.

I focus much on European history because, as a white American, these are my roots, but indigenous folk practices across the planet have always honored spirituality while allowing for strong women and sensitive men, for the self-selecting of gender expression, for love between same-sex or gendered persons to exist in peace. Cultures indigenous to North America, whose spiritual practices were so strong they were woven seamlessly into the practices of daily life, recognized two-spirit individuals, who seemed to carry within them the essence of both male and female energies. Yoruba, a spiritual practice indigenous to the Yoruba people of West Africa, inspires with its pantheon of gender-bending orishas, deities who, in the words of queer feminist writer and poet Moyomade Aladesuyi, "exist outside of our binaries." In indigenous Filipino spiritual practices, the shamanic babaylan roles were filled by strong women and gender-variant men. Even the briefest explorations of global pagan practices offer glaring evidence of how the white, puritanical culture that put witches to the stake across Europe spread their same violent, freedom-hating punishments across the globe via colonialism. The gifts that folk magic offer to people of color—especially queer people of color—are numberless, a reclaiming of wisdoms that threatened white settlers and their notions of white supremacy, female subordination, and capitalism.

Feminists and queers, women and elders, and people of color–is there anyone witchcraft *isn't* for? What about broke folks? As a kid growing up Catholic in a low-income enclave of New England, I sensed the hypocrisy of Jesus's support of poor people and the unfathomable riches the Church had stashed away across the globe, but especially in Vatican City. The whole hierarchy of the Church, from the Pope at the top all the way down to the middle-manager priests who were supposedly the only ones who could speak to the divine on my behalf, it all looked like a corporation, didn't it? And this was before we learned about the sexual abuse scandal the Catholic Co. *still* takes great, horrifying pains to cover up. In light of this, witchcraft offered me further empowerment and safety. In this disorganized and individual practice, I didn't have to pretend to believe in any human authority figure; I wasn't in danger of being manipulated by someone who supposedly had more access to the divine than me. In witchcraft, we all have equal access to the divine, and no one is getting rich off of it! I do love the fuss of lighting candles at my altar and using my little cauldron to burn herbs, but the truth is, my witchcraft would be every bit as legit and powerful if I simply walked into my front yard and struck up a conversation with the palm tree that lives there, perhaps snatching some fallen rose petals or sprigs of rosemary from the bushes that grow wild around my house, and leaving them at the grand palm's roots. Probably even more so.

In my tarot practice, where I read cards for a large clientele that spans the globe, in my work hosting and producing the acclaimed *Your Magic* podcast, and during the year I hosted a live, call-in tarot show, I have heard from *a lot* of witches who aren't quite sure they're witches. They *want* to be witches. They see it there, just beyond them—a magic practice that would be special, meaningful, inspiring. They don't quite know how to get there. I want you to know you don't have to become another person to step into a magic practice—you can step into it today, as you are, and tweak it all to suit who *you* are. Maybe you're someone like me who already has an established practice, someone who is constantly hungry for more contemporary takes on magic, new ideas to help us feel connected to magic in our time and place. *Modern Magic* will be the spark that sets your own magical practices buzzing.

THE BASICS OF MAGIC

There are more magical traditions, across history and today, than any book could do justice to—from earth-worshipping Wiccan or other pagan traditions that track the seasons; to the late-1800s, alchemy-inspired secret mystery schools, like Thelema or the Brotherhood of Light; to Satanism, with its dramatic symbolism and ceremony, which is having an American renaissance. What they all have in common is a belief in the un-known, that there is more to this world than what we see with our eyes. There is energy we can grab, to better our lives and the lives of others. The dead are perhaps with us. It is possible to know the unknowable, through intuition or psychic ability. Animals are vital. Earth is a literal, layered hunk of magic, spin-ning in an infinite vat of ever-more unknowable energy.

Sometimes, the notion that *everything is magic* feels liberating to me. I don't have to try so hard; what I need to be is observant, and grateful, conscious of the daily, easily overlooked moments of enchantment in my day, and present enough with them to conjure thankfulness for my life here on Earth. Other times, this feels like a cop-out, and I feel called to look to tradition and the tools of the spellcasting trade to bring my practice into focus. There's an ebb and flow of my own practice between these two points—a loungey, all-good, latent, hippie-witch magic and a more action-oriented practice that honors *my specific energy* and the things I want to manifest in my particular sphere. This feels natural to me, the middle path between magical sloth and high-pressure productivity.

BUILDING YOUR ALTAR

When I'm ready to get off my ass and practice, I go to my altar. An altar is really just a surface that holds your magical tools; it should be respected, and not share space with other, non-magical items. In this way you are creating a little spot of sacred space, which helps get your mind into the elevated state that responds to ritual. My own altar is the top shelf of a medium-size bookshelf. It sits in my office, which has a door I can close for some privacy if needed. Spellcasting and magic-making forces you to be vulnerable at times, to speak out loud or do a little dance, to pray or to meditate. These actions are most effectively performed without being interrupted by a nosy roommate, or lover.

I follow the tradition of honoring the elements with my altar. The recognition of the four primary elements on Earth is ancient, with water, air, earth, and fire—plus the heavenly aether, the fifth, ethereal element—being the building blocks of our reality. The elements are a recurring theme in many metaphysical practices. Not only do various pagan traditions honor them, but also we see them in action within the suits of the tarot, and the categorizing of astrological signs. (This repetition helps solidify the real-world, social, and energetic properties of the elements in your mind, and I will lay out these overlapping embodiments of the elements in the section that follows.)

EARTH: The earth element is the fertile, growth energy of the planet we live on. It's abundant, creative, hardworking. It's a bit goal-oriented, and also attuned to seasons—seasons of growth, of harvest, of loss. I generally use crystals to symbolize earth energy on my altar; they are made within the earth, via pressures and processes that continue to feel unfathomable to me. They are so varied, and so beautiful. Most magic is metaphor; I see in a crystal the beauty I might become or create if I apply consistent pressure to myself. I also can't ignore the wealth of belief systems that honor crystals as having their own properties: rose quartz helps boost your self love, amethyst stimulates intuition, etc. I do like arranging crystals on my altar in accord with something I'm trying to manifest—a successful project, a peaceful relationship, physical health, material wealth, a safe and sheltering home. We can ask them to help us harness the earthly powers of fortitude, solidity, discipline, and growth, to make something of our time on the planet, to leave a lasting mark, something to hand down once we reach our inevitable peak as ancestor.

AIR: With the element of air we ponder the mind. School, communication, knowledge, writing, metaphysical thought, philosophy—it's all in the realm of air. On my altar I enjoy using smoke; burnable herbs scent the air itself, rendering an invisible element temporarily graspable by one of our senses. Seeing smoke rising and carried upon the air acts as a great metaphor for rising thought, just as its tendency to drift away can help us take the compulsive, often harmful thinking of our monkey mind less seriously. I let bundles of herbs smolder in my cauldron; burn incense sticks bought at a church in Spain; or sprinkle loose herbs, or resins purchased at occult stores, onto a screen warmed by a candle to conjure smoke. Because the air element is historically represented by feathers and swords, I will sometimes place a found feather on my altar, as well as random sharp objects, such as the spine of a stingray found at a natural sciences shop, or the little plastic swords that spear a cocktail olive—it's good to be creative, and to have a sense of humor. In the tarot, air (frequently represented by swords) is infamous as being one of the bloodier, more painful suits: a comment on how we humans make our lives hard with our misunderstandings, our stinkin' thinkin', our mental confusion. Asian spiritual practices—Buddhism in particular—focus so heavily on taming the mind because there is a sense that all of our problems begin, and so can end, here. But there is delight and electricity in the air, too, as well as taste and discernment, the ability to imagine new futures, to push at the bounds of what is known, to embrace the unknowable.

FIRE: For the element of fire, I of course use candles. We see earth all around us, all day, water, too; we literally breathe air, but the relative rarity of experiencing fire in its raw element makes its presence feel instantly elevating. To have a bit of this powerful element—volatile enough to bring mammoth destruction—contained upon my altar is incredible, like having a miniature lion purring atop my bookshelf. As an element, fire represents, variously, our spirit or soul, our passion and ambition, our drive and our energy. It covers the sexy part of romance, the wildness of getting swept off your feet, the primal vibe of our feral sex drives. It also governs creativity, artmaking, and play. Fire covers a lot of bases, and because it is symbolic of our own personal energy field *and* our desire, fire comes into play in almost all of my spells. Fire means action, and every spell needs at least a little of that, if not a whole lot.

You can enhance the potency of your candles and their spells by dressing them—anointing them with oil, carving wishes or symbols into the wax, dusting them with herbs or glitter, sticking them with tiny stones. In this way, a candle can become representative of all the elements, and the complexity of your desire. In the tarot, the fire suit of wands, or torches, often illustrates victory, sometimes simply the triumph of being on the spiritual path that's right for you. Fire can take many forms, as we see in the fire signs of the zodiac—from the wild spark of flame that risks burning out or out of control; to the contained fire that nurtures a community; to the noble fire of expansive thought, which aims to illuminate nothing less than the human condition.

WATER: I choose to represent water on my altar with an actual vessel of water. Sometimes it's a teeny-weeny glass mug from my grandmother; or a goblet made of ornate black glass from the Madonna Inn, the place where I first acknowledged I was in love with my husband, and the place we eventually wed. Other times there's a fat jug of moon water, or a shimmering, iridescent seashell. Energy turns stale, and if you want your altar to be a living spot where you engage with yourself and with the numinous—rather than another shelf of dust-collecting knickknacks—you've got to switch it up. One reason I love having a goblet of water on my altar is that it evaporates, which pushes me to refill it, and to remain cognizant and caring of the sacred space. Water represents our emotional selves, and this is no big surprise when we think of the most obvious sign of high emotions: tears. Happy or tragic, we know we are feeling our emotions when the ocean that lives inside us spills out. Presumably, you know all about the benefits of crying—how our tears contain antibodies and minimize stress hormones, clear out toxins and rally endorphins. They regulate the emotions that provoked them to begin with, leaving you in a chiller state than when the sobbing began. The element of water, in magic, represents purification of the sort we receive from a good cry or bath or shower. It represents our tender hearts and the way they can be moved with joy or shattered with grief. It represents relationships, catalysts for all sorts of tears: love, commitment, friendships, family, and also heartbreak when any of these connections turn sour. Water is also mystical. It is where life on Earth originated, and individual humans *still* begin their existence immersed in fluid. It is moved (as are our moods) by the moon, and rules spaces which have no borders, where movement is easy and individuation moves to the background in favor of interconnectedness.

AETHER: There is, of course, a fifth element, the element of aether. A creation of antiquity, thought of during medieval times as the invisible force that filled up space itself, aether has come to mean many things in magic. Sometimes it is a stand-in for the life force, such as the Asian prana, or chi, an energy that is conducted through our body as well as throughout the cosmos. It can be read as the ineffable, the unknown, the great mystery, the divine. It is known as akasha in Sanskrit and The Force in *Star Wars*; it is the Void or Nothingness of Buddhism and, for alchemists, the missing ingredient to the elusive philosopher's stone. There are pagan traditions that encourage practitioners to represent this fifth element on their altar with a flower, an image of a deity, or even a mirror, to reflect their own divine nature back to them. For quite a while, I kept a thrift store knickknack on my altar, a ceramic unicorn with a chipped horn, draped in a little bracelet I had made while crafting with my son, beads that spell out Q-U-E-E-N-<3. I kept it there until I had to change it up; now it sits on my windowsill and is legit winking at me as I type this. On my altar, spirit is presently represented by a large, golden crown, its peaks ornamented with stars. I like to nestle a candle within it and watch as the flame shoots star-shaped shadows across my room. Aether is present in all the elements, and as such does not have specific astrological signs in its governance, nor a suit of its own within tarot. There is no magical tool that corresponds with it exactly, because it is what we use our tools to connect with and manipulate—the life force that all matter springs from.

With the elements represented and tended to on my altar, it's time to play with some spellcrafting. *Play*, actually, is the most powerful ingredient in a spell's efficacy. Numerous studies about the power of playfulness for adults have added science to this magical notion, correlating playfulness with increased excitement at being alive, decreased stress, and increased coping skills. When I set about casting a spell, I feel in touch with the little-kid version of myself, trying on new and different aspects of "self" and conjuring a big, wish-making imagination.

Is spellcasting wholly make-believe? No more or less than any spiritual practice. Because it delights me, helps me gain focus on my often nebulous desires, and triggers all the neurochemical rewards a state of play brings about, I have come to value spell-casting regardless of whether it "works." But, the reality is, it *does* work, often in strange, paradoxical ways, such as refusing you the things you wanted that weren't actually good for you. Sometimes, I believe that these little errands of fate are being run by entities from the spirit realm—a spirit guide who works alongside me, biological ancestors looking to help me live my best life, or even chosen ancestors, historical figures, or god-dexxes who I feel a kinship with, and whom I sometimes ask for help in spellwork. Another way I comprehend spellwork is to understand that the universe is filled with *energy*, currents of force and movement, that respond to intention. Like catching a wave and surfing it to shore, I sometimes envision a spell sending my wishes and desires out into space, where it syncs up with an energetic pulse that supercharges it, explodes it, and brings it home.

When we engage with spellwork we are really engaging with mystery—the wonder of life on this fertile, growing Earth, in our strange, fleshy, permeable bodies, brimming with imagination and desire. Witchery is a safe space to turn away from the wholly rational, to put the crown of primacy on feelings, emotion, intuition, play, and longing. We give thanks for the mystery and summon the true faith to launch our hopes and lusts out into the creative chaos, knowing that *we*—our bodies, our feelings, our energy—are also important aspects of the great unknown. We sync up with the great mystery, make a wish, and sit back to see what happens next. Whether you draw from tradition or make it up as you go along, modern magic is an inherently, and inspiringly, customizable practice. Here's to you finding your own ritual groove, whatever playful form it takes.

JUST FOR TODAY ALTAR

My participation in various 12-step groups brought me closer to magic. While a lot of folks who check out this world have their hackles raised by the *God*-y-ness of it all, I took to heart the promise that the higher power we're urged to seek is one of *our own understanding*. Never mind that I mostly do *not* understand what my higher power "is"—the Universe? Hekate? Stevie Nicks? *Me?*—I embraced the opportunity to dive deeper into the wonky magic practice I'd inconsistently nurtured. My personal drugs of choice had often been futile attempts to commune with the divine—the wine of Dionysus, the love and sex promised by Aphrodite!—so it made a certain sense that part of abandoning destructive intoxicants would be looking to connect with magic energies from the purity of my own body, mind, and spirit.

One of the many pieces of *content* 12-step practices deliver is a little prayer-poem-mantra-essay thing called *Just for Today*. Folks in recovery aren't the only ones who feel routinely overwhelmed by the world and their place within it. That's a human thing, and the intensity of feeling so overwhelmed only grows with the times. To whatever might be going on in our own lives at any point, we can add social media, climate change, and the chaos of late-stage capitalism to the mix. *Just for Today* offers us a moment to still ourselves, press pause on all that, and, rather than freaking out, align ourselves with The Now. We "fit ourselves" to the luck we've presently been granted, rather than bang ourselves up with the anxiety of striving. We pledge to, temporarily, "not find fault with anything." We dare to be momentarily "unafraid." It goes on and on. Talking about oneself actually brings on dopamine, a happy brain chemical in short supply among those swearing off anything, so it makes sense that 12-step writings tend to run on a bit. But therein also lies its charm: being advised by the program to "take what you want and leave the rest," we can scan the document and select what we might like this sacred, eternal moment to consist of.

In the following "spell," google to find a free pdf of Alcoholics Anonymous's *Just for Today*, and select three humble claims that appeal to you. Then, utilize the magical internet for a peek at where the moon is. What sign is it in? Get inspired by the zodiac sign and its element, and build yourself an altar to *NOW*. Bring something into your magical space that salutes the energies the moon is reflecting out at you, and grab something to honor the sun's energies as well. Is there a holiday vibe happening? Acknowledge any seasonal happenings, as well as any special days your traditions of origin or choice recognize. Maybe it's your birthday season, or there is a personal anniversary coming up? Allow those to be part of your NOW. The spirit of this action is one of gratitude, and of deep recognition. As the witchy Fever Ray song intones *Now's the only/time I know*, the same is eternally true for us all. In taking a moment to be at one with the fleeting present, you are syncing up with so many philosophies that urge us to give thanks to our swift and humble lives by just sitting, breathing, thanking. Meditate before your altar, or do a little dance—the choice is yours, and perhaps influenced by whatever is happening during your special moment in time.

While *Just for Today* aims to center us in the moment, we all know that every moment leads to every other. There is a sly edge to this writing in that it can become a practice of centering yourself in the Now, when the sky hasn't fallen, when you are relatively safe, when you can lean into the coziness of the moment and allow it to grow stronger, until it is a magical presence that helps ward off the *what-ifs* we hex ourselves with on the daily. Whether it grows into a balm for anxiety or simply a sweet moment of gratitude for what we've been gifted with—and whether your occasional altar stays random or blooms into something regular—it's always a simple step from the mundane into the magical that can shake some magic loose and reorient you toward your self and your beautiful life.

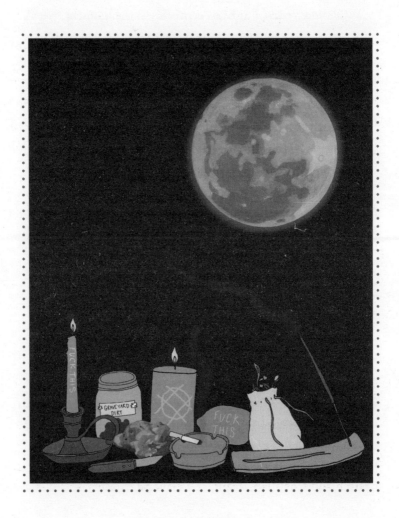

Welcome to
My Coven

The chapter title is a bit of a joke—I don't have a coven. Likely, neither do you. The majority of people interested in witchcraft and magic experiment with it on their own, picking up herbs and books at occult stores, lighting a candle, setting crystals out before the full moon. I started adopting these practices—burning incense or little tufts of dragon's blood, stuffing a satiny pouch full of flower petals and tying it to my leather jacket—in high school. High school, famously, is a drag. Alienated from the Catholicism of my youth, having taken up a wardrobe of thrift store widow's weeds and fallen in love with bands with names such as The Lords of the New Church and Christian Death, my elaborate strangeness was a

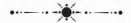

target in my homeland of the north shore of Massachusetts. Cars zoomed by, flinging trash and insults at me. I was spit at on the street, menaced on public transit. My family was distressed; why would I solicit all this negative attention? Did I have to dye my hair blue and color my lips black? Somewhat frightened, they were more understanding of the urge to pelt me with empty McDonald's wrappers than my urge to dress so dramatically. "I'm just being myself," I protested, demanding protection and understanding I did not get. It was okay. I got those from my friends, a group of similarly misunderstood goths fighting with their own families in 1980s Boston. One new friend, Gwen, even lived in Salem, where the witches were famously burned. All of New England feels haunted, but Salem especially so. The city danced a delicate tango, expressing regret for the murders associated with the famous hangings, while leaning into the spectacle for tourist dollars. The local cop cars had images of witches riding brooms on the doors, and the town honored longtime practioner Laurie Cabot as the Official Witch of Salem. Her shop, Crow Haven Corner, was the oldest occult store in the country, and she blessed the high school football team every year. Gwen liked to call her "the official bitch of Salem" after nearly being hit by her sleek, black car, but I always suspected she was lying; outcasts that we were, it was hard to embrace any authority figure, even the unlikely figure of a laureate witch.

I was never afraid to mess around with witchcraft. My nine years in Catholic school had the unintended effect of making me completely wise to the manipulative mythmaking of the church.

A virgin birth? Please. Sounded like fear of women's sexuality to me. An underground, flaming cesspool to house "sinners" for all eternity? Sounded like a great way to instill fear in the masses and bully them. I would have *liked* to believe in muscle-winged angels, and a sneaky, seductive Satan (and sometimes do!), but mostly it all struck me as fictional as the Greek pantheon of gods. Zeus probably wasn't hurling thunderbolts. God probably wasn't sitting on a cloud sussing me out like a sour Judge Judy. But there was *something*.

Like a lot of people who find their way to witchy world, I loved ghost stories and tales of the spirit realms. UFO tales gave me excited chills. Books about telekinesis and clairvoyance, ESP and "sixth senses" held me in thrall. Anything and everything that suggested there was more to physical reality than what we took for granted, more than the black and white, good and bad *borrrrring* morality of religion, filled me with a sort of energy. An inspiration. A *knowing*.

I didn't exactly know who or what I was directing my early, teenage magic toward. I was asking for things—boyfriends, mainly—but to whom was I proposing these requests? I wasn't sure. I enjoyed conjuring an out-of-focus, mystical goddess, a feminine energy that probably wasn't even embodied, that was maybe just a *vibe*; we only projected a physical body on her because that's what we know on earth—flesh, the material. In this source, I felt liberated to ask for fleshy, material things. My Catholic upbringing frowned upon praying to God for selfish things like toys and trips to Disneyland. But this way of worshipping, from what I saw in spellbooks, seemed to encourage a person to want things, and to ask for them. I wanted love, mostly, and I wanted a big, exciting life. I wanted to be strong in the face of my tumultuous home life, and I wanted to be both protected and brave in the face of the small-minded people who harassed me on the daily.

I've learned so much, and have watched the culture change, in the many years since I was that teenage goth girl, but I'm still her every time I approach my altar. I still don't exactly understand who or what I am offering to, only that it makes a certain, dormant part of my psyche come alive. As that part of me that needs and responds to spiritual things opens up, I feel calmer and inspired, connected to the great mystery of what we even are, where we are, what it all is. It's so agonizing down here sometimes, isn't it? But it's also so gorgeous, such a wonder. I ask for things—"success" (whatever that is), opportunity, hot sex, increased intuition, abundance, safety. And I offer gratitude for everything I amazingly, improbably have: a writing career, a skilled tarot practice, a really cool husband, an amazing child, lifelong friends, sobriety. I light candles and burn things that fill the room with fragrant smoke; I line up crystals and knickknacks on my altar (aka, the top of a bookshelf), and I spritz myself with water that sat under the full moon or slide a drop of witch-crafted tincture under my tongue. I meditate on a puffy *zafu,* bringing the years I spent sitting and studying at the San Francisco Zen Center into my practice. Sometimes I work with a *curandera* who prepares baths full of flowers and herbs that help cleanse me of the worldly bullshit that gunks up my vibe. Sometimes I order protective spritzes from a witch with a Romanian and Jewish practice, to help me maintain my boundaries and psychically safeguard me from the forces that *still* work against people who live outside the norm: witches and queers and trans folk, people of color in a white supremacist world, people with bodies and abilities that defy the ways we're taught a body should be.

I came to magic as an outsider, someone who had woken up to the ills of the world and could easily spot the glaring connections between the ways the world was treating me and the ways they treated these "others." I would continue to become more of an outsider throughout my life, as I embraced feminism and came out as queer, as my queerness evolved to bring me into alignment with trans people, as I made a living in the sex industry, as I realized and committed to the lifelong project of anti-racism, as I became the mother to another being on this Earth. All of these things brought me into deeper connection with the world, and brought me into greater conflict with so many of its people. And witchcraft is here for it.

What even *is* witchcraft? As someone of European descent, and who learned about it through trips to Salem, my own practice is pretty Eurocentric, bits of pagan that and Wicca this. Because I am not part of an established tradition—the notion is attractive and I'm a joiner! I've just never been asked—I have the liberty of making it up as I go along, winging it. What I have ended up with, after decades of practice, is a fully bespoke— couture, if you will—spiritual practice. I pull my inspiration from mythology and history, from pop culture and queer ancestry. I worship Hekate, the Greco-Roman, goth Queen of the Witches, and I also offer devotions to Flora, the Italian goddess of flowers, who captures the part of my spirit that feels forever youthful and optimistic and holds endless wonder for flowers and scent. I have at times felt drawn to Afro-Caribbean traditions, but wary of appropriating cultures not my own, I instead dove deep into my own Polish ancestry, and came to understand that *all* cultures had their own folk magic before Christianity came in and ruined the party. I reach back into my DNA and connect with Trishna, a goth Polish goddess who protects corpses and hangs out in cemeteries; Flora's Slavic counterpart Lada, a giddy May Queen; and sex goddess Zizilia. It was thrilling to understand that all of us, no matter who we are or what our ancestry, have a witchy tradition in our past, waiting to be discovered.

One of my favorite witches, the writer Vera Blossom, once advised me that, when confused or wary, the act of *asking* can be elevated to the level of a spell: "Rather than feeling paralyzed about accidentally invoking a deity you shouldn't, or summoning the evil eye by accidentally appropriating something from a cultural practice, approach practitioners and magic shops with questions, ask about a new spell, bring up what your needs are with other practitioners, and find something that feels right and true." Don't be afraid to admit that you don't know and need guidance! Humility is always a spiritual bona fide, no matter what your tradition.

While you're busy googling dieties and looking for practitoners to query, I would like to share with you some spells from my own history, recent and ancient.

MICHELLE'S FUCK THIS SPELL

Apologies for being so crude, but can't you just *feel* the magical power in such language? They're called *curse words* for a reason. One of the simplest and strongest magical tools at your disposal is your own voice. We take air, and we move it through our body, creating vibration. When you think of it like that, our words do seem like magical offerings, don't they?

For this spell we will channel the defiant *I've had it* of a teen. Perhaps you were not a defiant teen; perhaps you were too intimidated to say *hell, no*; or perhaps you were raised in an affirming space that gave you little reason to rebel. Regardless of whether you are/were a nervous nelly, were well-adjusted, or have a history as a disaffected youth, we all know the archetype of the wild child. If she wasn't you perhaps she was your friend, a specter at school who boldly challenged social mores, a character in a book or film. Whoever she may be, conjure her in your imagination. Sit silently and call to you a femme spirit of defiance. I imagine the Princess of Swords tarot card as illustrated by Lady Frieda Harris in the Thoth deck—hurling herself upwards on a cloud of fury, possessed of beauty and rage, dashing up at the sky with her sword drawn, as if prepared to tear down reality itself. And this spell is especially great when it *is* reality that needs to be resisted; when there is legislation being passed that threatens vulnerable communities; when groups of people as small-minded and angry as those who killed the witches are gathering in your community; when a group of humans is being singled out and scapegoated; when you yourself feel the sting of injustice in your life.

Gather some magical tools. I recommend a candle, a pin or sharp blade, pepper, a piece of citrus, and, if you happen to *already be in the habit of smoking things*, something you smoke (I recommend an herbal cigarette stuffed with flowers, if you can get your hands on it). You do *not* need to do this to successfully enact this ritual. But for those who do indulge in this particular vice—a vice that I, like many rebellious youths, picked up in my teens—do use it here. It may mean that you bring this ritual to an outside location, rather than stinking up your home. No problem. Outdoor magic is, in so many ways, preferable if you can swing it. Smoking witches should also have a food coloring pen—you know, those markers you can write on cupcakes with, available at many grocery and craft stores.

With your blade or pin, carve *FUCK THIS* into your candle. Set it down, and surround it with a ring of pepper. Light it. I chose pepper for its obvious repellent spiciness; it's an herb that packs punches, which you will be conjuring. It's associated with Mars, the Greco-Roman god of war and the planet that helps us handle conflict. It may be helpful for you to know what planet your own Mars is in, and see if that can help you further envision your personal rebellious teen deity.

Take your citrus, and likewise carve into the rind *FUCK THIS*. I chose citrus because, like life, citrus is sour and also sweet; we cringe against its flavor even as our mouth waters for it. While it's the sour sting and injustice of life on Earth that may inspire us to perform this ritual, we also must never lose sight of the mysterious beauty, the yummy pulp of our lives. Citrus goddesses include the Indian Alakshmi, a goddess who brings poverty and misfortune; and the Italian goddess Pomona, whose energy brings intoxicating blossoms to citrus trees and causes them to bear tangy fruit. It appears that humans have always recognized the sweet and sour metaphorical, magical properties of citrus.

Sit before your candle and fruit and think about that teenage goddexx you've conjured. Locate and observe your energy inside your body. Where can you feel it? The top of your head, burning in your chest, the tension in your face or shoulders? Take some breaths to both relax yourself and to gather that energy and send it throughout your body. Start to focus on your breath. With every in breath, think *FUCK;* with every out breath, *THIS*. Get a rhythm going. *FUCK. THIS. FUCK. THIS.* Imagine the people, places, or things that you wish to cast out of your energy field. A particularly evil politician? A family member who has done more harm than good? A certain repressive energy you have realized holds you back? What do you say to these forces? *FUCK. THIS.*

Please note that the mantra is not *fuck you*. This is not a curse or a hex. The *THIS* that is getting fucked (and to get fucked, I should mention, is in reality a wonderful thing; but for the sake of this spell we will lean into the word's properties of extreme refusal) is its power over you, be it the space it takes up in your brain or the fear it conjures in your heart. You are meant to live freely on this earth, and, in doing that, you always take risks. Are you risking the censure of these forces by being your amazing self? You are? Well, *FUCK THIS*. You're not going to let hateful people take up space in your brain or restrict your joyful movements.

I said earlier that speaking aloud is a powerful magic, one that uses the element of air and the holy flesh of your own body to create vibration. If you are in a place where it is safe to start chanting *FUCK THIS*, please do! You are issuing a literal vibration of resistance into the air! How cool!

And if you smoke a papery substance? Write *FUCK THIS* on it with your food pen, and smoke it, thinking *FUCK THIS* as you inhale and exhale. You're feeding your rebellious teenager deity as you smoke. Don't do it if you're going to feel guilty or yucky or sick; do it only if you can indulge it with a spirit of fierce, rebellious *FUCK THIS,* and send your message into the ether on puffs and plumes of smoke.

I think it's a good idea to take a nap after this ritual. Or do it at night and go to bed. You've pulled out some deep energies and have exorcised them in no uncertain way. Let your psyche process and your system reset. When you rise, know that your pissed-off teenage deity is in your heart, spurring you to take no shit and get on with your excellent life.

LADA FEMME SPELL

Lada is the Polish goddess of springtime and women. Like most goddesses, she was a boss bitch and actually had *many* realms to watch over, but spring/new beginnings was her signature vibe, and as she was a protectress of women, I believe she has the backs of all femme creatures, regardless of whatever sex/gender you've been assigned or are navigating.

I believe that femmes—people who express, cultivate, and run feminine energy—have particularly powerful magic. Sorry if that sounds reverse-sexist (JK, that's not a thing), but all you need to do is look back through time and space for evidence of the femme's connection to intuition, spirit realm, and magic generally. Even the least *woo* femme in the femme-dom still exudes a sort of charm (the root of that word is the Latin for "enchantment," by the way); it cannot be helped.

Maybe you want to grow your femme powers in how you express yourself (like, you want the courage/inspiration to *femme the fuck out*, visually speaking), or you are interested in strengthening your traditionally femme powers of intuition, divination, and other moon magics. Perhaps you are feeling haunted by the reality of violence femmes face on the daily, and you want extra protection. Whatever your need, Lada has got your back. First, choose a candle. Green is nice, as it honors her as the queen of spring, but pink also works, as a reclaiming of a hue that has been assigned to girls, therefore seen as weak, but is actually a fantastic color that radiates love and party vibes. Onto your candle, carve Lada's special symbol. It looks like an empty tic-tac-toe grid, tilted on its side, surrounded by a circle. It should form a diamond in its center, and the tips of the lines should extend through the circle. You can also carve it into a piece of fruit and either eat it or leave it as an offering, or, if you're so hardcore, scratch it or draw it on your skin. While you are doing this, speak to Lada, aloud or in your mind. Ask her for what you want: increased femme magic, strong femme protection, or both. Maybe you have a femme friend who is in a bad situation particular to femmes and you want to ask that Lada watch over her. Keep the spell alive by growing your relationship to Lada, by continuing to talk to her and meditate on her.

TRISHNA CEMETERY SPELL

Trishna is a minor goddess in the Polish pantheon, but as the patron of cemeteries she got my immediate attention. Like Trishna, I have always enjoyed the atmosphere of a graveyard. My grandparents lived across the street from a very old graveyard, and during the era I lived with them the spot was my playground, a green space in a city afflicted with urban blight, offering stones of chiseled beauty that put one into a contemplative mood about life and death and the mystery of it all. I broke my wrist riding a bike in that cemetery, and I had my first real kiss perched on a tomb. My husband proposed to me in the Hollywood Forever cemetery, site of our first, Covid-era date, where we roamed, masked and six feet apart, gazing at the final resting spots for Dee Dee Ramone, Vampira, and Mel Blanc (his grave reads: *That's all, folks!*).

Graveyard dirt—basically, ground soil from a cemetery, especially from the ground above a particular grave—has long been used in magic. From ancient Egypt to the American hoodoo practices originating with enslaved Africans, the combination of literal earth, with all its inherent energies of grounding and abundance, with the added oomph of proximity to one of our greatest mysteries, death, make graveyard dirt a potent magical tool. Add to it the energy of so many humans who have come to any grave site radiating love and grief, admiration and respect, and you have some extremely charged earth.

(Alright, I don't have to say this, do I? I'm going to say it anyway: when I say *graveyard dirt*, I mean a tiny scoop of earth from the ground. That's it! Don't go messing with actual *graves*, with stones or bones or plants or flowers, okay? *Thank you*.)

Such a sacred substance as graveyard dirt should be utilized for your most important spells. So first, what do you want? Creativity? Love? Power? Abundance? Money? Family? Once you've selected what you'll be casting for, do some research on your local cemetery. Who is buried there? Any known creative people? Surely some married couples, bound together in the hereafter. Any leaders, folks who had amassed power and abundance during their earthly lives? If you can match your desire to a person who in life had that same desire met, the dirt from their grave will have a special resonance.

Find the grave. If you have any trouble, don't be afraid to ask a cemetery worker for help. In my experience, they welcome human interaction, and enjoy showing folks around the place. Also, cemetery workers tend to like cemeteries, so they're not going to think you're a big weirdo for roaming the grounds.

When you are alone at the grave, speak to Trishna, guardian of this place. Tell her you come with pure heart and gratitude, and that you would like to take some earth to make magic. Tell her what you are seeking and why. Next, address the dead with pure heart and gratitude, and ask them the same. Of course, you are unlikely to hear *Go for it!* from the ether, but you will be able to feel in your body if it is a "go for it," or if it's a no-go. If you have any bad or yucky feelings, perhaps abort your mission. Sure, that wobbly feeling might just be your discomfort with being in a cemetery and digging some grave dirt, but if you're not comfy with such a ritual you shouldn't be doing it, anyway!

Take no more than a handful of dirt from the grave. Bring it to where you do your magic. I would put it in a jar or a cute little bowl, but if you want to just heap it on your altar, fine. It's your space, your magic. You can simply leave it there as an offering, something to meditate near before each day as you work to conjure what you want. You can include it in a larger ritual, ringing it around a candle in a color that corresponds with your desire, or get super playful with it and make a mud pie, replete with decorations of flower petals and stones. Graveyard magic—and graveyards!—need not be dour and spooky. In my Southern California home, local cemeteries are frequently sites for outdoor movie screenings, art exhibits, puppet shows, and community celebrations, such as the enormous Día de los Muertos festival that fills the Hollywood Forever cemetery with live music, food trucks, and tons of loving altars. Respect your graveyard dirt, and enjoy the rituals it inspires.

Patron Saints and
Other Witches

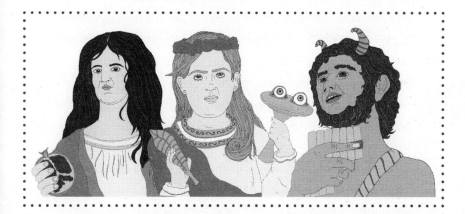

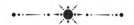

I often think that my desire to reach out toward some unknown energy larger than myself—through spellcasting, devotion, meditation, aligning myself with the history of witchy people who have come before me—is the most human thing about me. Our history is full of myths and religions and superstitions and rituals, gods and goddesses and all the many strange and beautiful things people have done to thank or appease them. Of course, many of these traditions have calcified through the ages, losing their mysticism and wonder and becoming little more than fear-based habits passed from generation to generation with little thought as to how they actually serve anyone. This might have been your early experience with "spirituality"—some type of religion with a pantheon and dogma you were told to believe in, and a handy mythological punishment awaiting you if you didn't. I've spent a lot of my life railing against such institutions and belief systems. But I also have found that, even in the most closed and dogmatic systems, there are the vestiges of mysticism: the possibility of something larger and beyond us. The romance of energies embodied in supernatural beings. The spellcasting, energy-manipulating, meditative power of prayer. If you peel back the messy chaos of most all spiritual traditions, what remains at the core is remarkably similar around the world.

My introduction to a spiritual practice was Catholicism. I suppose it could have been worse. Of all the branches of

Christianity, Catholicism retains the most of the pagan, indigenous folk magics it usurped and outlawed. Much has been written about the witchy, decidedly non-Christian roots of the big Christian holidays, but still I marvel at the audacity. Take Easter, the Christian holiday that honors the crucifixion and vanishing of Jesus Christ (who, for the record, seems like a way-cool dude, hanging with sex workers and preaching nonviolence, using his psychic powers to get wedding guests crunk). It occurs suspiciously close to the spring equinox, which was dedicated to the goddess Ostara in Eastern Europe. Clay "Easter eggs"—fanciful, colored, egg-shaped decorations—were found on the grounds of a medieval city and traced back to the tenth century. The onset of springtime, with its obvious connections to birth, renewal, and fertility, things olde pagans loved to throw a party about, was coopted by the Church, who slid their own deity neatly into the mythology with a convenient tale of "resurrection."

Same goes for Christmas. Centered around the winter solstice, the darkest night of the year, festivals that emphasize literal and metaphorical "light in the darkness" rule. You can imagine how magical an evergreen tree must have seemed, with its ability to stay green and lively year-round; how sweet to honor it with ornaments and candles, to even bring it inside the home, using sympathetic magic to help us make it through the longest night, the hard, cold winter. The solstice is the worst of it—after that night, the sun begins its slow path back to fullness and springtime. Swap out the sun for the son and behold the clever way the Church swiped this holiday as well. (And don't get me started about the reindeer goddess of the indigenous Sámi people of the Arctic, and the way Sámi shamans would observe the winter solstice by tossing psychedelic mushrooms down villagers' chimneys. Google it.)

As a child, I was awed and inspired—and, eventually, bored out of my gourd—by the interior of my local church. Our Lady of Assumption, a name fit for gags, was as garish and overdone as a Catholic church famously is, influencing my aesthetic for life with its velvet-lined altar, the golden chalice tucked inside a gleaming tabernacle, the outrageous bas-relief sculpture of heaven, replete with a bearded, white God stretching out toward us from a cloud. Second grade brought my first experience of true femme finery—drag, if you will—with the purchase of the fluffy white dress I would wear for my first communion. It came with a *veil*, and the veil came with a *tiara*, and I thought that I might *die*, it was so gorgeous. *I feel like a princess!* I distinctly remember gushing to my mom. Before you judge me, check your femme phobia. I refused to stop *werking* this outfit, even as we celebrated my taking of Eucharist with a trip to Benson's Wild Animal Farm. I dirtied my shiny white shoes in the crud and dust of the zoo, using my veil to filter the animal stinks away from my nose.

Lest I seem like I'm waxing too nostalgic about an entity that has done more harm to women, queer and trans people, and abuse survivors than any other *in the world*, let me apologize. I have no illusions about the violence and injustice the Catholic Church actively perpetuates, globally. I haven't gone to church since getting confirmed in eighth grade, something I tried to get out of doing, having recently discovered goth nihilism and panentheism. I wouldn't put a penny in their coffers. But it's tricky, just a tiny bit. Catholicism is the tradition where I discovered the goddess, and learned to pray. And praying is simply spellcasting, without the bells and whistles.

I was obsessed with Mary in middle school. As a young girl I intensely related to all girls, period. I still can't watch a film or a show that doesn't have a lot of femmes in it; I just tune out, leave my body. Images of femininity ground me, and Mary, who was represented by statues and portraits all over my school, had me in thrall. It felt special that I went to a school that was *named* for her, named for her holy and mystical ascension into Heaven—sort of like getting tractor-beamed onto the mothership, but, like, different.

For those not versed in the ridiculous tale of the Virgin Mary, let me hip you to the myth: Mary was a teenager, engaged to a dude named Joseph, but still a virgin. The angel Gabriel pops by her place one night, waking her up with his trumpet (rude) and telling her that, though she hasn't ever had sex, she's pregnant, and her baby will be the "son of God." This causes some friction with her and her fiancé, who is like, "Yeah, right." Gabriel swings by Joseph's and is like, "No, dude, for real," and everything is chill.

I've had lots of thoughts about this myth through the years. It's formative for me, having been given a goddess at such a young age, and it is lodged in my psyche. As a queer person who went through much toil and trouble to birth my own son of god, I'd love to believe in the errant instance of immaculate conception; how great it would be if those who had uteruses could spontaneously reproduce, like a whiptail lizard. But, as this has never been seen IRL, it is clearly a myth. Or, a lie. What if Mary had cheated on her fiancé, and, being an impressively imaginative person (as well as a skilled actress), convinced her man of this mystical occurrence? In a darker vein, what if she'd been raped, and wished not to have the insult of misogyny added to the injury of her attack? What if, in either scenario, she had to keep up with the ruse, raising her baby to believe he was some sort of messiah, making him the patient zero of messiah complexes? What if she suffered a mental illness that created delusions? There are lots of scenarios to imagine, but the one where she's knocked up by God feels about as probable as the goddess Athena bursting from Zeus's thigh.

These intellectual exercises were alien to me when I was a child dazzled by my first goddess. In second grade. What really kept me enraptured was how it was supposed to happen *again*. There would be a second coming of Jesus—all the Catholics were stoked about this ancient promise. But, if there was going to be a new Jesus, that meant there would have to be a new Mary. And I wanted it to be *me*.

I felt I was in a vague but enormous competition with literally every other girl on the planet. I could feel the eyes of God upon me——I felt that anyway, was raised to feel it—sussing me out as the potential Best Girl Ever, the one best suited to birth round two of the messiah. I believed I was a contender. I was *good*. I did well in school, didn't fight with my sister too bad, mostly listened to my parents. As the realization that I maybe *was* in the running to be the Earth's Next Top Virgin Birther sunk in, I began to monitor my behavior more intensely. I did *not* want to *fuck it up*.

But I did. My teacher, Ms. Poiree (who was nearly fired for incredulously asking a class of seven-year-olds, "You still believe in the Easter bunny?"), handed back a quiz one morning, and my little belly lurched and dropped when I saw that I had gotten *a bad grade*. A bad grade? A bad grade! Bad grades weren't *good*. It meant you hadn't studied or were an idiot, and you can bet that peeping God up there in the sky didn't want the mother of his next holy child to be some lazy dumbass. I knew—I *knew*—that somewhere in the great big world was a girl who had not gotten a poor mark on a quiz that day. She had done well, and, congratulations!, was still in the running. Not me. I was out.

I slid the test under my regulation cardigan sweater and asked if I could go to the bathroom. Down in the cold basement, in the empty girls' room, I tore the test into a hundred pieces and fluttered them into the trash can. I destroyed the evidence. I wouldn't talk to my parents about it, and maybe I would, eventually, forget about it. But guess who never would? Who saw and judged everything, all the time? God. I let go of my desire to be the next Virgin Mother of God. But I never really let go of Mary—the first of many iterations of the Divine Feminine to trigger that devotional urge in my spirit.

It's precisely its inclusion of Mary in its pantheon that makes the Catholic Church so different from other strains of Christianity. She is the pagan goddess kidnapped and appropriated, so that worshippers could still hold on to their femme devotion while being manhandled into a new belief system. Ancient and even modern churches still show evidence of this, retaining pagan details such as gorgeous rose windows, which honor the goddess, or outrageous Sheela Na Gigs, the decorative hags holding open their giant vaginas that decorate the outside of old European churches; Ireland alone boasts one hundred of these wild dames.

I think my predilection for devotion stems from my time in the Church with Mary. Warned to never pray for material things, I was hesitant to ask for anything, and my prayers tended toward gratitude: that my family and I were safe, had food, were healthy. Though I thought Jesus was fine, from a young age I felt uncomfortable around men (moody, alcoholic father, perhaps?) but loved female energy, and felt intuitively connected to Mary. The idea that she would watch over me, like a mother, made sense. I gave myself to her, directed my nighttime prayers to her, fell asleep feeling held by her.

As I became a teenager I turned against Mary, just as I turned against everything about the Catholic Church. *Obviously,* the Church crafted her a virgin birth because they all hated women and couldn't deal with lady parts and the powerful mysteries of their bodies (this read still stands). Having gone goth and witchy, I cast about for other deities to worship. I considered Satan, as one does when rebelling against the Church. The transgressive shock value alone is pretty worth it. I found a copy of Anton LaVey's *The Satanic Bible* at Newbury Comics and made a purchase. It was great fun to read on the subway; my giant, spidery hair and deathly pallor were already going to draw unwanted attention, but *The Satanic Bible* struck fear into the hearts of many in this Catholic region. They whispered about me, but mostly left me alone.

Aside from being a protective shield, I found *The Satanic Bible* surprisingly cool. In the author's hands, Satan was just a cool, rebellious guy who dared speak truth to power. More a symbol than an embodied entity, to be Satanic was to be a free thinker, a libertine, nonjudgmental, sexual, living for the moment. A persecuted teenager looking forward to growing up and getting the hell out of New England and into my wild and liberated life, I approved of Satanism, and loved to explain to anyone who would listen how misunderstood Satanists were. They didn't want to drink your baby's blood; they just wanted to cosplay and have orgies! Still, though I was down with their cause, it didn't quite capture my mystical attention powerfully enough to draw me in. Probably all the dudes.

My understanding of my Catholic heritage shifted powerfully with the introduction of a *botánica* in my city, on a little street by the bridge that led to Boston. Botánicas are occult stores specifically for practitioners of Afro-Caribbean magical traditions: Santería, Yoruba, Ifa, Espiritismo. As a teenager I had already discovered more Wiccan-oriented occult stores, such as Crow Haven Corner in Salem or Arsenic and Old Lace in Cambridge. The botánicas *felt* like these places, spots of heightened energy that made me feel dreamy as I stepped through their doors. The things they sold were similar, but also very, very different. There were oils, and herbs, but also soaps and sprays. There were candles, but rather than being poured into plain jars, the glass was marked with images and prayers, in English and Spanish, to various deities and entities. Including, to my surprise, a whole bunch of Catholic saints.

There was Saint Lucy, with her eyes on a plate. Saint Barbara, with her chunky crown. Saint Rita, her third eye shot up with the holy spirit. I even spotted Jesus—baby Jesus in his dapper representation as the *Nino de Atocha*—and multiple Marys, her dresses fat, her halos extravagant, holding her baby and stepping lightly on clouds, or water, or the crescent moon. I had never seen the icons of my family's religion represented in an occult fashion, and I was transfixed. Through books I came to understand how Africans kidnapped from their homes and forced into slavery on islands colonized by Europe hid their beloved and banned deities behind the images of the Catholic saints being shoved down their throats. And so Saint Rita, the patron saint of the impossible (especially impossibly shitty relationships), stood in for Oba, who rules marriage, and was the first wife of the god Chango. Chango, a super-manly god, was represented by Saint Barbara, as they both ruled fire and lightning. The Nino de Atocha, with his feathered hat and shepherd's crook, his capelet and ruff (swoon), was known to be Elegua, a charming trickster god often seen as a child. And on it went, as did my understanding of a *syncretized* spiritual practice.

I was inspired by the creativity and devotion of these enslaved African people in the Caribbean. I began to see Mary and the assorted Catholic saints (whose grisly martyrdom both attracted and repelled me) not as who the Church said they were, but as whoever I wanted, or needed, them to be. As a sober adult in a 12-step program, I learned the phrase, *Take what you like and leave the rest.* Intuitively, I began to apply this to the icons of my youth. When I lit the candles I purchased from the botánica, I was not petitioning Virgen de la Caridad del Cobre, the Virgin Mary as Our Lady of Charity; neither was I venerating Oshun, the Yoruban love goddess. I saw both deities within her, but also, she was the ancient goddess, pre-Christian, worshipped globally in the image of the people who loved her; she was the generative power of the universe, maybe the universe itself. She was the great mystery, capable of everything, and as I set my candle burning on my dresser—unknowingly creating an altar—I asked for things. A boyfriend, surely and sadly, but also protection and abundance, and I felt gratitude well up in me as I recognized how, in some form or another, pieces of what I longed for were already available to me in my life.

I once heard the writer Elizabeth Harper refer to herself as "culturally Catholic," and I felt something click inside me. While this identity is not exactly at the forefront of my spirituality, or who I imagine myself to be, with that phrase I suddenly felt a little space open up within me for this problematic and nostalgic, grisly and gorgeous, complicated tradition. I imagine that many of us who stray from the traditions we were born into—especially those who stray toward more mystical practices—do find a way to sneak back and grab whatever rituals and icons we feel are ripe for reclaiming. As for me, at this point, Mary is so embedded in my concept of the Goddexx, there's no extracting her. The saints, the female ones, light up my shadow self, my internal Persephone, the way my psyche has eroticized pain and suffering, sacrifice and femininity. Agatha of Sicily holding her breasts on a platter, like little princess cakes; Saint Teresa, her ecstasy so perfectly articulated in the sculpture by Bernini you can practically hear her moan; Lucy, with those creepy eyes of hers on that little tray. I can't turn away from these tortured, fascinating icons. And, thanks to the syncretic nature of witch-craft, I don't have to.

I AM MY OWN GODDEXX

This is a spell to amp up your own divine vibes, and increase your understanding of your self as Goddexx, made in her marvelous image. It's meant to stimulate that part of your self that has a direct line to the cosmos—maybe even the corner of your psyche that understands you (we) *are* the Goddexx, creating this reality as we go.

It is a pagan practice to place a mirror on your altar, using your own self to represent spirit, the Goddexx, the divine. So, def do that. I love that. Get your altar going—light your fires, spritz your spritzes, whatever it is you do to let yourself and the ether know that you have *arrived*. And once you have arrived, sit down and begin to meditate. Center yourself. Feel and ac-knowledge your body, acknowledge and flick away any rando thoughts that pop into your mind (so annoying, but they're just doing their job). Once you feel settled into yourself, think about who you would be if you were a goddexx. Are there certain aspects of your personality that stand out strongly to you? Can you locate those strengths in other deities? Want to borrow something from them? Can you encapsulate your strengths in a metaphorical object or color your Goddexx displays, or a landscape where they are situated? Perhaps there are passions and interests that define a part of you, and you want to bring those into the image of your divine self. Maybe there are animals you relate to deeply—give yourself some ears, a tail, scales, wings. Maybe there are flowers, or crystals, that super resonate, and you want them to be part of this portrait.

When you feel like you've conjured a complete-enough image of your inner divinity, journal about it. Draw it, if you're talented like that (or even if you're not). Add to it as you go, as inspiration hits. Do you name this deity? Give them your name, or a secret name that belongs to you? What are they the goddexx *of*? If others were to petition them, what would they ask for? What type of offerings do they (you) enjoy? Set some of it on your altar. What is their color? Light a candle in that hue. Where we often seek to see ourselves represented in a magical image, here we have located the magic within, and crafted the image around it. Worship yourself, ask yourself for a wild dream to come true, and see how you deliver.

A SPELL FOR SAINT TERESA

I have a religious knickknack of Saint Teresa that I found at a thrift store. A small, wooden triptych, the center panel depicts the Spanish nun with her head flung back, her arms outstretched, her body washed in a gorgeous, golden glow. This saint is known for her religious ecstasies, but in this, and most, representations of her, she looks lost in a much more physical bliss.

The Church assigned this lusty, mystical saint to watch over sick people, chess players, and lace makers. But clearly, she is available to those who want to infuse their mysticism with some sensual bliss, as well as those who would like to bring a mystical edge to their physical pleasures. For this spell, you have permission to move your altar to your bedside, or create a bedside mini-altar, or just lie on the floor before your normal altar, and masturbate. But, wait! First, you ought to grace your magical space with an image of Saint Teresa, light a purple candle (red, too, if you have one), and grab any amethyst and carnelian stones you might have. Purple is the color of psychic ability and intuition, and amethyst corresponds with that. Carnelian is lusty; once I took a nap with a smooth, tumbled ball of it in my underwear, then woke up and went on a pretty mind-blowing sex date (TMI?). Anyway, you are to have a mind-blowing sex date with yourself, right now. As you light your candle and arrange your altar, ask Saint Teresa to help you bring magic into your pleasure, and pleasure into your magic. Let her know you intend to have a transcendental orgasm. She can relate, and is rooting for you! Now, masturbate however you normally like to except no porn or erotica (sorry); toys are cool (always). Think whatever thoughts do it for you, but see if you can't intersperse it with a mystical element. If you're a heavy fantasy person, weave occult magic into your story; if you're a purely physical beast, understand that you are also making contact with powerful cosmic energy, not just your junk. At the moment of orgasm, send your energy out from your body with intention. While sex magic (that's what you're doing!) is a practice that allows you to ask for/manifest anything, in this instance you're going to intend for this orgasm to help you get closer to the divine. A brighter vibe, stronger aura, sharper psychic abilities, super-charged intuition, a sense of extreme closeness with the Goddexx. Something like that. Afterwards, take a nap if you can. When you wake up, journal about your dreams immediately.

A SPELL FOR SAINT LUCY

Saint Lucy is depicted with her eyes on a platter to represent her martyrdom by the gouging of her eyes. Yikes. In these depictions, Lucy *also* has eyes inside her head, to spare us her grisly reality. Her enucleation has made her the patroness of blind folk, as well as one who watches over martyrs. We all would have been wise to make offerings to her in the early 2020s, as she rules over epidemics as well as infection of the throat. She also looks after salespeople, and—yes!—writers! Feel free to seek her out when you have a cold or are working on commission, but right here I'm going to devise a spell—I mean, a prayer . . . I mean a spell . . . oh, same thing!—to help those who, like me, struggle to get words onto the blank page or that blank, glowing screen.

It's interesting that a saint without eyes was selected to watch over writers. Though the sighted among us do, of course, use our vision to get the words out, what is most important in writing is that *inner eye*, the imagination, the mental ability to link words together, link concepts to concepts, link phenomena in metaphor. It's our *mind's eye* that writes our writing, and I can attest to our physical eyes being a true detriment to our literary progress. It's my eyeballs that look upon my writing and deem it trash or useless, derivative or cringe. It's in the rereading—that breaking of the creative flow to judge my efforts—that my eyes land on phrases and progressions that deflate me, fill me with frustration, push me out of the chair and off in search of a stress-reducing snack. Yes, Saint Lucy, poke out these orbs, so that I may stop laying the evil eye on my creative projects!

Um, no, wait, wait! We don't want to ask Saint Lucy to remove our eyeballs—how literal! But we can make an offering to her, as writers, that she watch over our efforts, keep us true to our own spirit and inspiration, keep our thoughts and words energized, focused, and flowing, and—most important—that she remove that evil eye from our mind. As a writing teacher, I always tell the writers I work with not to edit while you're writing. Writing and editing are two great tastes that *do not* taste great together. Now, I understand that writing processes vary, and there are some writers who can effortlessly edit while writing without it breaking their flow or giving them an existential crisis. If this is you, huzzah! Move along. For the rest of us, it does seem that writing and editing come from two different parts of the brain, and editing, with its necessarily critical eye, is too harsh to unleash during writing time, when you're in a more subconscious, imaginative, and vulnerable space. Saint Lucy, with her special understanding of vision and blindness, dullness and illumination, is a fantastic patron for those of us who especially want to keep the piercing gaze of judgment off our writing so we can get our lackluster first drafts out of our heads and, later, sit down and spiff them up.

For this spell, done best at your actual writing space, right before you get to work, bring an image of Saint Lucy, a yellow or orange candle, and, if you have it, some honey calcite (Great for writing!). Also, if you have any silly eyeballs left over from Halloween rolling around, you can include those, too (why not?). Light the candle and ask Saint Lucy to keep your inner eye wide open to inspiration, to give it steady focus and bring you into *flow*. Or, feel free to ask her for whatever writing-related favor you're needing, including for a big advance. Saint Lucy watches over *writers*, not writing, and writers need to be taken care of. When you remove the Catholic iconography from its Christian roots, as we have, the admonishment against asking for betterment in the material realm is *gone*. This is the realm of the Goddexx, the cosmic energy that built the universe. Ask for that six-figure deal! If she can, Saint Lucy will make it happen.

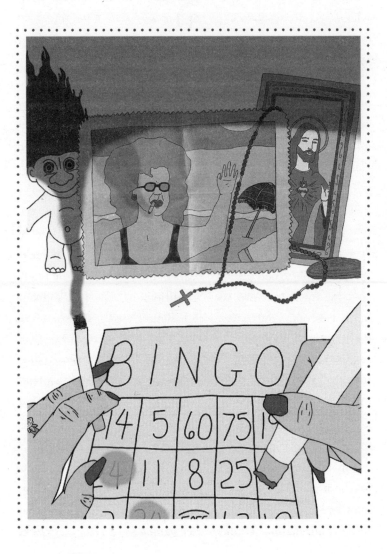

Luck, Good and Bad

The women of my family were very serious about luck. When I turned eighteen years old, they deemed me ready for initiation into their tradition. My mother and her mother escorted me to a church basement. It was all women in there, mostly older women, elders. Each had assembled an altar of sorts before her—little dolls, photos, pressed flowers, coins. Rosary beads, prayer cards. And, between each woman and her little altar were sheets of paper stamped with rows and rows of sacred numbers. The air was filled with smoke. The mood was tense, very anticipatory as we waited for the ritual to begin.

I'm talking about bingo. I got so hooked that first night. Maybe it was the nicotine-fogged air that got my heart racing, but there is something about the *possibility* of a bingo game that revs my adrenaline. Unlike other gambles—poker, blackjack,

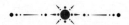

slot machines—with bingo, *someone* is going to win. It could be any of us. Why not me? Why not you? As a preternatural optimist, bingo appealed to my deep belief that everyone's a winner, that life works out, that anyone can have a lucky day. And that night, it was me.

It's a very intense experience, calling bingo. I was not ready for the strong, occult energy in the room to be immediately focused on me, to hear tables of elder women spit, "Shit!" while full of glares and grumbles. "You're lucky," my grandmother said, a benediction that washed away the bad vibes of my jealous comrades. Seventy-five dollars is always welcome, especially when you're an eighteen-year-old working at a crappy convenience store. But what was truly valuable was the feeling of being ushered into this activity that was part fun and games and part prayer session. Because, even though *someone* was going to win, the fact that it was *me*, in this superstitious, highly Catholic crowd, meant something special about me. For other potential winners in the room it would mean that the Christian God was looking down on them, that Jesus had their back. But for me, and the women in my family—Catholic for show, but off-gassing the pagan vibes of their pre-Christian, European roots—winning meant we were linked to the ineffable. We were touched. We were magic.

I would tend to think luck was just a made-up concept, if not for one strange day in Las Vegas, when I woke up feeling "lucky." What did it feel like to feel lucky, you might ask? It felt a little sparkly. It felt fresh, a sort of brisk cleanliness. At the time, I was none of those things. Just off a month-long punk performance tour in which I encountered all-new alcoholic lows, I'd cheated on my girlfriend and was awash with guilt. When said girlfriend came to pick me up at the end of the tour, I was sickened in my body, mind, and soul. I cried fat, dramatic tears as we drove back home, from Chicago to San Francisco, tears that glowed electric blue from my mascara, plonking down on the tin cans of beer I nursed in the front seat, scrunched down low in my girlfriend's vintage Ford Falcon, hiding from cops. I'd quit my job to go on tour, and so I was flat broke. It was my girlfriend who paid for the gas to get us home, the food and hotels along the way, and the sorry cans of beer I guzzled. My dependence on her, and her uncomplaining acceptance of it, only fueled my misery.

That in the midst of this pity party I woke up feeling "lucky" is mysterious. I shuffled my Thoth deck and pulled the ten of pentacles, titled Wealth in this tarot. If you think pulling the Wealth card in Vegas is a positive omen, you are right. My ex/girlfriend and I both had a love for Vegas's wild, trashy excess, and we decided to stay the night. We joined a bingo game at the now-demolished Frontier Casino, a joint with a Western vibe. I promptly won $75. We took my winnings to The World's Largest Gift Shop, where I tried to buy some guilt reduction by showering my ex/girlfriend with tacky gifts. We put the remainder of my purse on another round of bingo at a different long-gone casino, the Mardi-Gras themed Showboat. There I called bingo again, but not just a regular bingo. This time I won the Powerball Jackpot, a $1,600 prize, enough money to pay back my ex/girlfriend for all she'd spent on me, as well as set myself up at home while I looked for another job. Sixteen hundred dollars went far in down-and-out 1990s San Francisco.

Back at home, I broke up with my girlfriend for good and began a seven-year, dysfunctional, yet also passionate, relationship with my tour fling. I also started a regular underground bingo game in my living room, replicating the Powerball Jackpot that I scored in Vegas. Every Thursday night my apartment would be filled with cigarette smoke, everyone's lucky tchotchkes bumbled before them on the coffee table, or where they sat cross-legged on my dirty living room floor. Everyone's inner bitchy old lady came out as they furiously blotted their cards with daubers, grumbling aloud that the numbers they wanted hadn't been called, cursing those whose cards were fuller than their own. It was fun for a while, but to be honest, I won too often for my friends' liking. As the bingo caller and the host of the game night, it seemed a little suspicious. When I eventually won the Powerball Jackpot, I feared they were going to drag me off to the guillotine. "I can't help that I'm lucky!" I protested, though a look around my life might suggest otherwise—my shower, for instance, was a tin closet, the floor rotted through in a rusty hole, yet the drain still completely clogged so that one had to wear water shoes *and* stand on a milk carton when washing oneself. Still, I knew that my proclamation was true. I *was* lucky. I still am.

It is easy to believe, when I win at bingo, that my nana, and also my great-aunt Ella, are with me somehow, watching over, using these games of chance to communicate their presence to me. One afternoon, as I played bingo at the kitchen table with my young son, he threatened to quit the game because I just kept winning. "It's because of my grandmother," I told him. "And maybe my aunt. You should make an offering to them. Maybe they'll help you, too." Game for a new activity, he acquiesced. We went upstairs, where I keep a small altar on top of a bookshelf and also a rolling cart of shelves stuffed with all the tools of my worshipful trade: sticks of palo santo, jars of dried sage gifted by friends, jars of protection incense, jars of dried lavender, mysterious jars of herbs I forgot to label (witches love a jar), and more. I gathered a little of this and that, plunked some crystals on my altar, and lit candles. I rang a little bell I had hung on a nail above the shrine, and spoke out loud. "Nana, and Auntie Ella, if you're here, this is your great-grandson and great-great-nephew. He has an offering for you, that you might help him improve his bingo game." I nodded at my son. "What are you going to do for them?" I asked.

My son stepped into the center of the room and proceeded to do the most wiggly, wild, unabashed dance. His arms were akimbo, high above his head and then waving out to his sides. He spun this way and that. His legs went up. He sashayed across the wooden floor. Out of breath, he finally stopped, making a flourish with his hands. "That was incredible," I said, totally impressed. Never had I made such a bold, spontaneous, physical offering to the Universe! My son had made the purest offering ever, an offering of his unique spirit, impossible for anyone to replicate. We went downstairs and resumed our bingo game. He lost. I won.

Is luck real? Is anything? Scientists can't definitively say we're *not* living in a computer simulation. Life is an enormous mystery—the hows and whys of our existence, what happens when we die—every part of our earthly existence is a puzzle that can break your brain if you try too hard to sort it out. I love magic because it allows me to accept the unfathomable unknowable *as is*. It gives me a template for worship and gratitude that feels good to me, that seems to elevate my humble office, for a moment, into a temple of the ages. I like feeling connected to a history of humanity that always had the urge to do *this*, to seek the great mystery and adore it. To make offerings of our small human desires, to beseech unseen powers to help us, to catch an invisible ribbon of energy and ride it like a surfer does a wave, straight to the shore of our best lives. I think luck is one of those waves we can sometimes catch, and I have created some spells, charms, rituals, and practices to help you catch it.

In any endeavor, in the pursuit of all desires, luck is one component. It can fill in gaps left by a lack of experience, a thinness of talent, a distracted nature. Luck is always present, and so luck spells can be utilized in any area of life: love, career, art, friendship, money, travel, you name it. Of course, sometimes they seem not to work, like my son's offering to his ancestors. Sure, it could mean that the whole thing is phony-baloney. Then again, in the grand scheme of things, perhaps it is far *luckier* to not get what you're wanting. Who knows? When dealing with the ineffable, we're always in touch with the big mysteries of our lives. Make the offering, do the spell, and then step back and let the Great Unknown do its job.

Dip your toes into the waters of luck-conjuring with some easy inspo from my son, and my favorite ex-girlfriend. In the fashion of my kid, make an offering to whatever or whomever you think could be lending a benevolent ear. Your higher power? The great energies of the Universe? You dear departed grandma? No matter your focus, call out to the recipient, and then do please dance your goofy heart out. Magic has no use for embarrassment or shame; like an actor in their most crucial role or a lover in the heat of passion, you must believe in what you're doing, what you're offering, with all your heart, mind, sinew, and sweat. Dance it out, and collapse on the floor. Offer gratitude for your ability to move in whatever way you moved. See what happens.

How can I justify the energy I put into standing before my humble bookshelf altar, lighting candles and *vibing?* I console myself with this: to make ritual is profoundly, biologically human. Anthropologist Dimitris Xygalatas arrived at this conclusion in his book, *Ritual: How Seemingly Senseless Acts Make Life Worth Living.* Speaking to NPR's Ari Shapiro, he asserted that rituals "help individuals through their anxieties, [help them] connect to one another. They help people find meaning in their lives." Our brains are wired to facilitate these types of meaning-making activities. Dr. Andrew Newberg is a trailblazer in the field of neurotheology, which studies how spiritual experience is shown in our brains. His brain scans of people in the throes of spiritual experience, from Pentecostals yapping in tongues to Tibetan Buddhists in a meditative state, illuminate how various regions of our physical mind are ready to fall back or rev up to help facilitate a mystical encounter. Prayers, chanting, and mantras—all repetitions of language—engage the frontal lobes of the brain, stimulating a hyper-focus. For folks in the process of channeling a spirit, the frontal lobes fade and the thalamus, the switchboard of communication between your body and your brain, lights up with activity.

Somehow, just knowing that my spellcasting and prayer, my superstition and my meditating has a traceable effect on my brain is enough for me. I can feel something happening—it feels good. Like Xygalatas writes, it helps me find meaning. I can write a story about what that meaning *is*—call it the goddess Hecate or the great god Pan, hope that it's the spirit of my grandparents popping in to say hi, or just call it *energy* and leave it at that. All that matters, for me, is I'm a human enacting what seems to be an ancient and crucial aspect of human experience.

Luck, in the world of magic, is a form of energy—a current in the Universe, a stream of sugared stars one can pluck with intent and ritual and heavy wishing. Of course, it also has a darker twin, *bad luck*, a stream of cosmic influence we surely never want to splash around in. Just as good luck might be harnessed by ritual, so might an errant, accidental, or even unknown movement unintentionally spill some of that bad stuff down on our hopes and dreams. In fact, many "luck" spells might more truthfully be classified as bad-luck-banishing spells, as they don't so much try to magnetize the good vibes as repel rotten fortune.

Think of the evil eye, the aesthetically pleasing, unblinking blue orb that is ubiquitous across so much of the planet, from Asia to South America, the Middle East to Europe, your text messages and social media comments, worn on chains and strings as jewelry, hung from cords in homes and businesses and vehicles, dangling in clumps from trees, like gorgeous, cobalt-blue leaves. Along with the lacy, elegant hamsa amulet—the hand-shaped talisman of Africa and the Middle East—evil eyes repel bad energy, in particular the envious or malicious vibes flung your way by other humans. With an origin in the Greco-Roman era, when the color blue was seen as a talisman of great power, able to ward off bad vibes, evil eyes were meant to assist the most prosperous of people, folks who lucked out with a hearty inheritance, a pretty face, or an envious marriage; word on the street was, getting too much praise could not only go to your head, it could attract hate from the masses *and* annoy the gods and goddesses. In the 300s BC, being afflicted with the evil eye was at least as prevalent as anxiety is today, and the symptoms were much the same: physical distress, mental anguish, having a hand in your own undoing. Physicians, unable to ascertain the root of a malady, would chalk it up to the evil eye.

Let's say that energy is a real thing, and that we all have it coursing through our body. When we're in a good mood we have light, bright energy. Bad moods stir up moody, rough storms of energy, like an angry sea. No doubt you have felt your energy influence other people, your cheer contagious, your gloom killing the vibe. Certainly, you have felt touched by another's happiness, and been brought low by someone else's bad day. This is just Life 101. Take it a little further, into the mystical (or paranoid) realm, and it's not hard to imagine how the bitter, jealous glare of a frenemy could have an actual effect on your well-being, killing a winning streak, smearing a cloud across your sunshine. Are we really all so powerful? Psychology would probably say it's an inside job; the thought of another harboring ugly feelings toward you, rooting for your failure, might make you nervous, self-conscious, defensive, or angry. With these low vibes running amok, self-sabotage wouldn't be a surprise, whether the distracting new fear causes you to mess up, or a subconscious desire to be less threatening causes you to demote yourself. Someone with a bit of an obsessive nature (heeeeeey!) might find themselves dwelling on the drama, indulging arguments in their mind, draining loved ones with endless, circular complaints.

I have no doubt that much (all?) magic will eventually be attributed to psychology, neurology, and other glamours of science; to me, this in no way diminishes or disproves magic's power. A rose by any other name would smell as sweet, and all that; if it works, it works.

Does wearing the glass evil eye charm actually repel yucky vibes? I can't answer that, but that didn't stop me from picking up an evil eye—glassy and smooth, satisfying to hold in the palm of my hand—after my front door got pelted by a dozen eggs. It was fucking aggravating, as it was near impossible to scrub off. I took that evil eye and I hung it from the lock on a window in my office, so that it glared out at the street below. When I worked at my desk in front of that window, I would look up, catch a glimpse of the soothing blue caught in a beam of sunlight, and smile. I felt like I'd installed a psychic security system on my property, and nobody ever egged the house again. After keeping it in the window for a few years, I finally removed it and began wearing it as a necklace. The weighty feeling of it around my neck, the way it sits so solid on my sternum, *does* make me feel safe. It's a good feeling.

Of course, I can't end this musing on luck without mentioning that I am in possession of one of the biggest Bad Luck curses in all of history: a female body. There is a reason Jewish men are encouraged to thank their creator for *not* having been born with a uterus and a vulva and a couple of teats. Now, if you are in fact trans, and made less-than-happy by the presence of these things, I get it. But otherwise, what is so luckless about this physical form? It hearkens back to the medieval belief that all women were witches—or, at the very least, were uniformly vulnerable to the corrupting influence of the dark arts. In various cultures, it is bad luck for a pregnant woman to attend ceremonies such as weddings or funerals; people shedding their uterine lining are banned from saunas, forbidden to cross sources of water, or even be around the general community. Even a female who is neither bleeding nor gestating life is often forbidden to touch fishing rods or join men on fishing expeditions, as their inherent bad luck will spoil the catch. There are bazillions of such rando superstitions the world over: a lady popping by for a visit on New Year's Day is bad luck! A woman on a *ship* is bad luck! Meeting an elder female in the early morning, bad luck! Christian cultures blame Eve, but these fears pop up absolutely everywhere. And hatred and fear of women, cis and trans, continues to fuel violence and repression today. What is a girl to do?

All I know is that fear is power: if my body has been regarded as terrifically evil for centuries, then surely it has the
same energetic charge as any crystal or talisman. How excellent
to know that, should I be running short on magical supplies, my
very own body is a cursing machine! In fact, if you would like
to sprinkle some super bad luck on a malevolent creep in your
vicinity, take a coin and give it a little rub on your vulva (or
upper thigh if you're feeling shy). Then, slide the coin, somehow, onto your victim's person. The coin has been effortlessly
hexed with your powerful femme magic, and will troll your
mark with its unrelenting bad luck. This is an especially potent
spell to cast on someone guilty of being abusive to a partner. In
the late 1800s, Bridget Cleary, an Irish woman, was murdered
by her husband, who was obsessed with the idea that she was
not herself, but a witch or fairy changeling who had stolen the
real Bridget away and taken her place. After surviving an era
of abuse by her deranged husband, Bridget was accused by her
cousin Johanna of rubbing a coin suchly on her body, and handing it to her as a curse. This reignited her husband's delusions
that the woman was in fact a fairy imposter, and, while locked
in a room with her, he set her on fire, as her family beat against
the door screaming, "'tis Bridgie!"

In our modern times, one way to honor and avenge the
femmes who paid with their lives and their bodies for the fear
and superstition of violent men is to say *yes* to our magnificent
and terrible power—our sensitivity to the ephemeral, the way
we magnetize energy and pull raw knowledge into us with invisible tendrils. We can avenge them by being the witches, the

fairy changelings, that they were accused of being. By brushing coins against the bits of our bodies that awe them, and then tossing them toward the real monsters. By pulling the good luck down to enhance the lives of those we love, and sending scowling eyefuls of evil at those who would do any of us harm. Whether we want to up our bingo game or intimidate an abuser, seek support from our ancestors or purge our own bad vibes, protect ourselves from envy or get some money, the magic of our physical form can help us summon luck or conjure a hex. Just think, our bodies are made of *seven billion billion billion* atoms (more or less, LOL), all of them vibrating with energy. That's *you*. Magic is summoning the currents we are made of, and sending them out to the great fertile and lucky unknown.

Here's some inspo for your own urges to lasso some luck.

A BIRD FOR JOHANN GEORG HOHMAN

Johann Georg Hohman was, by trade, a printer, a bookseller, and a witch. A European settler in Reading, Pennsylvania, Hohman brought with him Germanic folk-magic traditions that had persevered from the Middle Ages, not only providing mystic healings and other magical services, but teaching others how to work with herbs and charms. This practice took root in Amish country as Braucherei. In 1820, Hohman published *The Long Lost Friend,* a grimoire that details these Pennsylvania Dutch magical practices. With remedies for toothaches, spells to ward off "wicked or malicious persons," and a ritual to win at gaming involving the heart of a bat, Hohman's book hearkens back to a time when physical ailments and human problems were all solved with magic. His influence on American magical practices is deep and legendary, and we will honor it with this Pennsylvania Dutch hex for luck.

Draw a star on a piece of paper: four-, five-, six-, or eight-pointed. In either two or four corners of the paper, draw a bird. Color it with primary colors, emphasizing green. Bring this with you when you gamble, game, or otherwise try to get some money. Braucherei—the name for the regional folk magic Hohman documented—is best known for the cheerful, geometric hex signs painted on barns and elsewhere throughout the area. The word *hex* derives from the German word *Hexe*, meaning "witch." In these artful hex signs, stars represent luck, as do birds; green represents abundance. Some hex signs sport stars with an impressive sixteen points; if your need for luck feels so urgent, please go for it!

LUCKY BAG

Get yourself a little cloth pouch. Fill it up with stuff that feels lucky, charged, or meaningful to you—a crystal or rock, a dried flower, a little toy, a picture, a piece of jewelry. Add to it some objects that have been infused with luck for centuries— some common and ancient good luck charms include acorns, dice, ladybugs, a wishbone, a hangman's rope, a nub of bamboo, a crocodile tooth. When your bag is full, sit with it before your altar and talk to it in your mind. Tell it that it's your Lucky Bag, and that you love it and appreciate it and that you know it's going to bring good things and positive vibes to you. Keep your lucky bag on you as often as you can, in a pocket or pocketbook or man-purse; pull it out when you really need to channel that luck! This practice is inspired by American Bingo superstition, as well as the African American hoodoo tradition of gris-gris bags, small flannel bags stuffed with stones, herbs, oil, sticks, roots, spices, bones, and personal items; like a spell, they can be created with any intention.

JOB'S TEARS

If creating a bag feels too fussy but you really want to ward off the bad luck, simply get your hands on some Job's tears. Otherwise known as Chinese pearl barley or adlay millet, these seeds are the grain of an ornamental grass native to Southeast Asia. Because the seeds naturally have holes in them, they have long been used as beads, in necklaces, on crafts, and to decorate clothes (a practice that began in India and spread out across the globe). In American hoodoo especially, the seeds are respected as powerful protective and wish-granting talismans. You can find them via occult shops online, which sell them for magic, *or* you can just buy yourself a bag of the grain. Simply carry three of them on your person to ward off malevolence—though I always like to take a moment to bond with my materials, say hello and thank you, etc., too. If you want to go a little further, you can string a necklace of the beads, and, since they're edible, you can also prepare them as you would rice and *really* metabolize their bad-luck-banishing power.

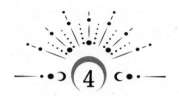

Divine!

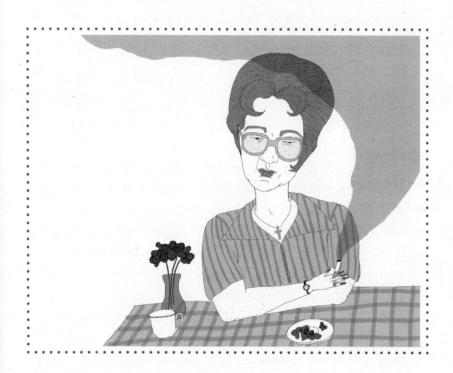

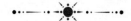

On that fated summer day in 1984, when my grandmother led me onto the city bus that took us over the bridge and into Boston, who knew it was a day that would determine the course of my life? Hopping from the bus to the Green Line, the subway blasting with heat from the screeching trains, the ancient grime sticking to our skin, I didn't know it. I was excited to be going into Boston—the big city!—so much more open-minded, cultured, and full of surprises than my hometown of Chelsea. The only surprises in Chelsea came from a boy running up behind you and smacking you on the head. And really, should you be surprised? Such violence was to be expected. In Boston, no one would smack me, and once I saw a woman with *green hair*, wearing a *cape*, shopping for tchotchkes in Faneuil Hall. Who knew what else I'd see that day?

What I was to see was somehow both mundane and more exotic than spotting a punk rocker. Getting off the train at Park Street, I could smell history in the burning electricity that traveled the mysterious tunnels. Up and out to the bustling Boston Common, the teeming shopping district anchored by department stores was too fancy for us. We would maybe hit Filene's Basement, where women my nana's age came to blows over the wooden bins heaped with deeply discounted items, and we would certainly hit Woolworth's for a hot dog and a Coke at the lunch counter. But rather than lead me down the cobblestone streets to these familiar haunts, Nana pulled me into a nondescript doorway on a side street. The tight lobby had barely enough room for both of us to wait for the elevator. Once inside the metal box, Nana hit number four and up, up, up we zoomed. When the doors clanked open, we were smack in the middle of what looked to be a rather humdrum cafeteria.

An elderly lady came toward us, older than Nana, who was only about fifty or so, though her polyester pants with the elastic waist, the hair she pin-curled each night, her drawn-on eyebrows, and her oversized eyeglasses did signify her membership to a bygone era. The older woman led us to a plain table in this exceptionally plain . . . coffee shop? At these stark little tables, individuals sat sipping hot drinks, and the air smelled like my kitchen at home, the dark, sweet odor of the Tetley tea my mother drank throughout the day. And this was what my grandmother ordered, a cup of tea. "One for the young one?" the elder waitress asked, and my grandmother shook her head quickly, with a bit of alarm, as if such a thing would be unheard of.

"Nana, what is this place?" I whispered, though there wasn't much need for silence. The room, with its white walls and high ceilings, sunlight blaring in through bare windows, was *loud*, ringing with the sounds of spoons clinking on china, cups clattering into saucers, and an unintelligible but constant stream of voices.

"It's a tearoom," my grandmother explained. "A psychic tearoom. They tell your fortune." I looked around, stunned. Fortune tellers, in this bland environment? Card tables ornamented with dusty plastic flowers in a chipped vase, stooped

New England matrons waiting the tables—this was where magic happened? Where were the glamorous women with jangling jewelry and dramatic makeup? Where were the velvet tapestries, the gold-leaf paintings of inscrutable occult symbols? The only things on the wall, besides a list of tea prices, were an old calendar featuring a simpering kitten and some curling newspaper clippings. This place was way too bright for the *mysteries of the unknown* to reveal themselves! And yet, as my nana received her cup of tea, I could see in her movements, in her expression, a sort of reverence; it was the way I comported myself during the first few Catholic masses of the year—open, somber, respectful—before boredom set in and my resolve to remain poised and holy disintegrated into fidgety annoyance.

Nana showed me the hot stew steaming in her fluted china. Unlike the soggy bags I was accustomed to, this cup of tea was thick with chunky, glossy leaves, a real swamp in a cup. My grandmother sipped daintily, only occasionally getting a leaf stuck in her lipstick. My grandmother's lipstick, pinkish and bright, ringed the teacup as it ringed the filters of the cigarettes she smoked, as it smeared my cheek when she peppered me with kisses. Like me, she was an Aquarius. She wore gauzy scarves tied around her hair, which I lifted from her dresser to knot around my neck like a disco dancer, or place atop my head, veiling my face like a secret princess. Her jewelry box was wooden, the drawers lined with velvet, and inside lay gold necklaces with clasps too complicated to work; these, these, too, were laid upon my head like slinky crowns. My little sister, with the deathless naivete of children, had called dibs on

Nana's engagement ring when she died, but I coveted a cluster of polished, pastel stones that could be *lifted* to reveal a tiny clock beneath! This was my nana, a regular New England grandma who worked the register at a local department store, put great stock in her dream life, and squirreled her granddaughter to a psychic tearoom hidden atop the shops of Boston.

That day, Nana got the most big-deal psychic in the joint, a large and seemingly ancient woman with great gray curls of hair and a palpable oddness. A squint at the walls revealed that the brittle newsprint clippings were all about her—her work with police in missing persons' cases, personality profiles. She was the tearoom's in-house celebrity. She joined us at our table and instructed my grandmother to stir the mucky leaves three times, clockwise, then tip the cup upside-down on the saucer. My nana did, and reverently. "Put your right hand on the cup and make a wish," she was instructed. Nana's hand rested briefly on the china, her chunky amethyst ring glinting. The psychic flipped the cup and peered at the clusters of wet leaves, looking for shapes and symbols that gave hints of what was to come. She saw letters: C, that was her husband, and her son; T was her daughter. The psychic spotted an airplane in the mosaic and told my grandmother that she would fly on a plane, but Nana never did.

"It's just for fun," my grandmother said in a hushed and nervous tone as we descended in the elevator. We were soon back on the normal, hot streets of summertime Boston, headed for the familiarity of Woolworth's, the easy din of shoppers riding the escalator, the simple fizz of a soda. "Don't tell anyone we did that," she urged. "The Church doesn't believe in it." My grand-mother managed the friction between her inner witch and her Christian upbringing by indulging her natural Aquarian interest in all things psychic, followed by a swift denial of any belief or seriousness. It was just a smidge of naughty fun—surely, we won't go to *hell* for it, but let's not let the townspeople know, lest they hang us for witchcraft.

Of course I told everyone—my mother, my sister, the kids at school—about my trip to the tearoom. The boys scoffed but the girls were intrigued, and the simple sharing of my visit pulled forth all kinds of stories: aunts who'd seen ghosts, TV shows about reincarnation. The boys rolled their eyes, but stuck close, listening in. The start of a pattern I'd witness again and again, the willingness of females and femmes to allow for the possibility of magic, and the longing for such a freedom all pent up in the chests of boys and men, straight and cis ones, any-way, as if they, too, wanted to believe, but aligning themselves with something so bewitchingly feminine, the unknown, was too much.

So, how did the trip to the tearoom alter my life? Well, even though that particular psychic didn't seem at the top of her game that day, I learned that psychic readings were a service you could pay for—a skill you could acquire, a job you could have. Soon I started sneaking into Boston and visiting the tea-room with friends, relishing their astonishment at such a place, the confusing combination of dreary and glamorous. Obsessed with the identity of the extremely goth boy—leather pants, spider hair—who worked the olden elevator at the record store around the corner, I wished on my overturned tea cup that I might learn his name. "Your wish will come true very soon," the psychic told me. In less than an hour, flipping through the Local Bands bin, I spotted him on the cover of an album by a band called The Blackjacks, looking tough, holding his guitar in a junky alley. The name on the back said Raphael. Raphael! Like the archangel!

Early in my freshman year, I'd hopped the bus after school and gone exploring in Boston in my silly, plaid Catholic school uniform. As the bus approached the public library, I gazed, astonished, at the clusters of kids hanging out on the wide cement steps. Weirdo teenagers such as the one I was in process of becoming, with my teased hair and black lipstick. Goth kids, punk kids, some looking like eccentric artists, some with skateboards launching themselves down the stairs, startling the commuters heading for the subway. I would become friends with all of them, in particular a spiky-haired boy named Peter who wore blue contact lenses and a padlocked chain around his neck. He was tough but soft, a new way for a boy to be, and a vibe I kept detecting in these new friends, boys with thrift-store trench coats and eyeliner smudged around their lashes. It would be a while before they came out, to me, at least, but these safe and spooky boys became my closest friends, Peter most of all.

Together we discovered tarot, the Rider-Waite deck first, and, later, the Thoth deck. That these cards both held magic and extracted from us our own inherent magic was clear. We slept with them beneath our pillows and thrifted silk scarves to keep them wrapped in. How did we learn of this tarot-maintenance lore, in the era before the internet? It must have been the hours we spent inside occult bookstores, studying, reading, hardly ever buying anything (though I did eventually acquire volumes one and two of *The Modern Witch's Spellbook*). From the moment I had my first deck, tarot became a constant, daily part of my life.

As my identity and my life shifted, so did my tarot. The closest I ever got to being a hippie was when I chased a girlfriend to the Arizona desert, and aligned myself with her vegan, anti-plastic, let's-live-off-the-land ethos. A fellow traveler reading cards in the streets of downtown Tucson introduced me to the Secret Dakini Oracle, a collage-art deck at once gorgeous and nightmarish, which drew on Tibetan mysticism that revealed the Christian limits of the Rider-Waite. Traditional tarot, with its strict declarations of meaning, seemed almost *rational* next to the wide-open mysticism of the Oracle, a deck I like to work with on new and full moons.

As my lesbian feminism continued to radicalize in ways that both hurt and healed me, I found the Daughters of the Moon tarot deck at my local women's bookstore. Glossy, purple orbs marked with a single crescent moon, the cards were multi-cultural and all-female; in their thirst for inclusion, they even created an optional male card, for those straight ladies who had not yet evolved into lesbianism. Titled "Pan," this nonthreatening man, skipping along a hillside with some children, did such a disservice to the lusty, drunken, big-cocked goat god of yore that I just couldn't work with it. Though I was at the time flirting with the extremes of political lesbianism, I still had a soft spot for Pan. However, I did love the flagrantly gay Lovers card—wherein a naked, biracial couple embrace before an enormous, radiant vulva—and chose it over the alternative Lovers card, which featured a biracial couple of indeterminate gender swimming to one another in a coral reef, sea plants handily hiding their genitalia.

I didn't set out to be a professional tarot reader, but when I landed at Peter's place in San Francisco a year or so later, newly heartbroken and scrawny with veganism, I located it as the one skill I actually had. My years of high school vocational training in "graphic arts" were useless; even if I had paid attention, the machinery was already outdated, everything gone computer. Writing wasn't something I could make money on, and besides, I probably sucked! But tarot reading . . . I remembered the hippie boy flipping cards for cash in Tucson. I knew my decks at least as well as he knew his. And so, following in the footsteps of the woman who read my grandmother's tea leaves what felt like a lifetime ago, I became a professional diviner.

Since then, I've read cards on the street for pocket change, spare cigarettes, and advice on how to get food stamps. I've read in shops and in my home. During the pandemic, my readings went virtual, and they've mostly stayed there, teaching me that the energy that makes the tarot work isn't exactly physical— the querent's hands needn't touch the cards—but something else, something more mysterious, ethereal, and powerful. I read tarot live on social media, or at charity events, at performances, at bars. There isn't anywhere the tarot can't go; people are always hungry for insight. Through these times and places, I've learned that this is what the tarot is best at offering, at least in my hands: insight. Yes, the cards can offer a peek into the future, which makes me think that such prophetic reads are actually a deeper form of the insight we gain from pondering our lives. Like, if we only pushed a little harder, relaxed our minds or honed our intuition, we all could see our futures, or at least an outline of them.

Tarot cards, and other forms of divination, trigger intuition through their use of imagery, and strengthen your intuition, so that you can access it even without the cards. Not that that is my goal—I love the tarot, and working with material objects is very grounding to psychic energy. I really value the thing-ness of tarot, and I also love the often playful artistry. In reading for so long I've come to really revere the tarot—it's so ancient, yet it can be reinterpreted into an infinity of contemporary worlds! And it *works!* Though I've been reading cards now for over thirty years, I frequently find myself gushing to clients, "Ohmygod! Tarot is real!" So blown away I am, again and again, by the ancient technology's uncanny accuracy.

Though leaning on my tarot skills was a crucial way for me to begin to financially support myself in San Francisco, it also brought me a possibly greater resource: community. The dyke-centric queer scene I encountered in the city's Mission District is now legendary, and for good reason. Lesbians and queer women seemed to rule the town, running all the best dance clubs, fronting the wildest punk bands, helming the hottest hangouts and filling the streets with swagger. I wanted to be best friends and girlfriends with everyone I saw. It was very overwhelming. I'm not shy, per se, but how to approach a mohawked stranger with shining facial piercings and armfuls of tattoos in a bar blasting Hole and Bikini Kill? Why, you walk up to them with your lesbian tarot deck and ask them if they want to pick a card! I promise you, they always do. While it might sound like a party trick, it's actually a way to get pretty real pretty quickly: If someone picks a triumphant card, you hear all about their latest big win, and you bond in the shared happiness of the moment. If the card is a bummer, you show up with compassion and sympathy. The reality of a painful situation showing up in the tarot lends problems a somewhat cosmic air, too. Maybe if this shit show is fated, there is meaning to be gleaned from it? Tarot elevates all of our lives by lending it metaphysical glamour, reflecting our movements in archetypal images. I made a lot of friends this way, and became somewhat known for being handy with a deck of cards.

And not just tarot cards. It doesn't take much playing around with the oracle to recognize its similarity to playing cards. Tracing the numbers one through ten, matching the four suits to the elemental quadrants of the minor arcana, you can talk about the layers of someone's life with the old deck of Bicycle cards crammed in the junk drawer, which I often found myself doing at parties when my services were requested but I hadn't brought my deck. One infamous night I even blew a seeker's mind with a spot-on fortune told with a deck of Uno cards! The same one-through-ten numbers combined with colors assigned, again, the elemental suits, and voilà! A blue four becomes Four of Cups, and you're mired in unquenchable yearning. A yellow Green and there's work to be done. Those "draw four" and reversal cards? I imagined them as setbacks and changes of fortune, respectively. It was such a fun project, I wanted to shift my divinatory focus to the game for a moment. It also helped me realize that *anything*— everything—can be a divinatory tool. You only need to assign the parts their meaning, and introduce randomness.

As divination had become my go-to salve for social anxiety, I sought it out upon finding myself at a birthday party for my most favorite writer, a poet I adored, was obsessed with. I say *found myself*, but really, I had learned an acquaintance had scored a casual invite to the gathering for the out-of-town writer, and I immediately glued myself to her side, determined not to miss this. While no one really cared that I'd crashed the party, I felt deeply awkward. The attendees were all generations older than me, had known one another forever. They traded gossip about people I'd never know, and shared missives from stages of life I couldn't imagine myself reaching. Home ownership? Child-rearing? How foreign and bizarre! I sat mutely, nothing to offer, trying not to gawk at the poet. This would not do! Spying bins of kiddie toys around the space, figurines in particular, I began to make some rounds, gathering them into an empty potato chip bowl. And then I approached the revelers, asking if they would like a "toy divination." Of course they would. I cannot stress this enough: *nobody says no to a divination.* Closing their eyes as I instructed, they plunged their hand into the greasy snack bowl and pulled out a Sesame Street character, a McDonald's figurine, a tiny superhero. Mostly, I recognized these characters, but for the ones I didn't, their costumes offered much information. Were they glamorous or clowny? Did they look evil, or animalistic? I zoomed in on each figure and "read" their vibe to the guest, attempting to make it say something about their own presence, or personality. It was a big hit. Even the ones who mumbled a skeptical "I don't know . . ." still seemed a little tickled by the game.

In the years to come, I'll be celebrating the first birthday of a friend's baby, and get to witness a *doljabi*, a Korean custom wherein a tray laden with meaningful objects is presented to the babe, and everyone waits with bated breath to see what item is chosen. The belief is the selection predicts the child's future occupation, and so the objects—a toy hammer, an airplane, a rope, a pencil, a calculator, a judge's gavel, a cellphone, a bow, a mixture of traditional and updated items—all suggest various professions. The child picked the airplane, and everyone clapped. Would he be a pilot? A traveler of sorts? The similarity of this eighteeenth-century practice to my little party trick gave me a sweet feeling. This urge to know, the belief that we can imbue the things around us with significance—or, maybe, suss out their essence—and use them to know more about our own lives, this seems to be deeply, beautifully human.

Recently, in New Orleans, I visited a Jackson Square psychic who offered bone readings. This woman was a hoodoo practitioner, knowledgeable in the mystical tradition that originated with enslaved African people adapting their indigenous pantheon and modes of worship to the brutal world they'd been abducted into. Like all Black arts, hoodoo has rooted itself deeply in American culture; while the practice seems more open—accessible to all—than closed, it is imperative that anyone engaging with hoodoo traditions absolutely give all glory and respect to the Black individuals, cultures, and legacies that shaped these rich and accessible practices. White people, proceed humbly here. One way to move forward is to pay a Black hoodoo practitioner for their services.

Bone divination is not solely African, or African American, in origin. Indigenous North Americans engaged in bone reading, or *osteomancy*, if you want to put on airs. Ancient archeological sites in central China have revealed the use of sacred bones. My reader's practice almost surely originated in Africa. Some bone-throwing traditions include other small objects such as dice, dominoes, shells, or tiny tchotchkes, and this conjurer kept some cowrie shells—revered for their connection to the feminine, and water—in her clutch of bones. She gathered them in her long, manicured hands, and had me place my own hands on top. After a moment, she let the bones drop onto the table below.

There are different traditions for casting the bones; circles marked with chalk or printed upon specialized cloth can designate areas ascribed with their own meaning. Some folks read the bones left to right, like a story. This practitioner gazed at the tumble of calcium and started talking. She told me I needed supplements, a lot of supplements. She actually named which ones would be best, but it was hard to hear over the brass band that had started up nearby. I am sheepish to say I did not take her advice—why get divination if you're not going to listen? Huh? Huh?—and nearly one year later, to the day, a doctor diagnosed me as deficient in vitamin B12, vitamin D, selenium, and a host of other minerals crucial to a functioning thyroid. Dammit!

The conjurer also pointed one long nail at a rather stubby,

phallic-looking bone and said, "You need more dick." I burst out laughing and looked over to see if my husband had heard over the blare of the horns; he had not. We actually have a pretty ferocious sex life but, to be fair, I am never satisfied, and on that particular trip I was promoting a new book, dashing all over the South, and we were frequently too beat at the close of the day to get it on. Huh. Like the conjurer herself, my husband is trans, and I wondered if what she was seeing in the reading was an absence of cisgendered dick in my life? Because we believed in her powers, we worked to translate her proclamation to my life. It ended in a shrug. "I guess you're going to have to give me even more dick," I smiled.

YOKO ONO TREASURE TOTE

W hy Yoko Ono? As the Earth deity sings in "Yes, I'm a Witch": *Yes, I'm a witch, I'm a bitch / I don't care what you say / My voice is real, my voice is truth / I don't fit in your ways.* "We women are all witches," she once said in an interview with *Vanity Fair.* "Witches are magical people." She's expressed this notion again and again, claiming the word *witch* in a way that is so easy and true, and inspiring many of us who *feel* we are witches but who allow imposter syndrome to stop us from wearing that proud mantle. Once, when traveling with John Lennon, she made a special trip to Salem, Massachusetts, to pay her respects to the women and the witches. Yoko Ono's own magical workings are evident in all of her art—her singing has the zawołanie power of mystical chants and commands; her writing and text-centric art often take the forms of impossible, mystical commands, directions for dream-time spellcasting. Surely the entirety of her artistic output could be gathered up and used as the raw material for a divination deck, cards with instructions, meditations, quotes, and sketches that the querent meditates upon. But that is a project for another witch, or at least another day! In honor of the playfulness and whimsy that attends her work, I instead offer you the Yoko Ono Treasure Tote, a divination technique.

This divination project can be ongoing. It is a mash-up of conjure bone-throwing, which does include nonskeletal items, and the toy divination that saved me from social anxiety at that party so long ago. Grab a bag—it doesn't *have* to be a tote, but if your house is anything like mine it is simply *brimming* in branded tote bags. Put one to use!

Next, you want to fill that bag with small, meaningful items. What makes an item meaningful? Well, this is a very personal endeavor. If you can see a meaning, a symbol, in the item, then it works. One idea: dice, which can mean a change of fortune or taking a risk; they're handily marked with numbers, which can carry their own meanings. Also, keys are small and loaded with historical symbolism. An earring might symbolize femininity, or the shape of it could mean something else entirely. Obviously, crystals come with prescribed powers, and you can include shells, bones (of course), and small plastic figurines: cars, animals, mythical characters. Junk shops and thrift stores are great places to find such things, as are natural science stores and the types of quirky, playful shops that offer little bins of plastic baby dolls and those monsters you jam atop a pencil. In short, absolutely anything goes, so long as all items are roughly of similar size. When your collection is smaller, you can shake the bag and dump the goods, deciding in the way they fall how to gather meaning. As your collection grows, and really anytime, you can give the bag a tumble and blindly select a single object, reading significance into what was randomly chosen. Such a mode of divination is extra-special, because even if a wild oracle bag craze were to hit us, and everyone was building a bag of sacred items, all bags would be different—and so you have for yourself a truly one-of-a-kind divination tool of your own creation. And I leave you with this bit from Yoko: "Everybody's an artist. Everybody's God. It's just that they're inhibited."

FLIP A COIN

Allow me to elevate the most mundane of activities into one of high magic. I give you: the humble penny. I personally will use no other coin in a decision-making coin flip; pennies are the perfect size, the perfect weight, and I admire their copper sheen. On the window ledge before which I am typing now sits a little decorative bowl filled with pennies; the piles of coins around it are pennies flipped, choices selected. I have a thrifted little dish on my bedroom dresser also filled with coins. I am a dedicated flipper of pennies, and I think you should be, too!

Of course, if you just *know* what you want, are sure of what to do, a penny is not for you! I admit, I too am sometimes so decisive! But, blame it on my sun and Mercury in the seventh house of ambivalence, I more often than not have a hard time making a choice. I can see the good and the bad in everything. Or, maybe I do know what I want, but it's the same thing I always want, and I'm wondering if I need to shake things up. The randomness of the penny flip is connected to the randomness of the universe, the randomness that fills our daily lives. Of course, chaos theory suggests that even in the most tangled and seemingly random phenomena there is an underlying order; it's an unproven theory, but it *feels* right, doesn't it? By introducing the chaotic flip of a penny, I aim to align myself with a higher, more mysterious ungraspable structure. Sure, it's a lot of pressure to put on the decision of where to eat dinner, but *I am a spiritual being having a human experience!*

An extra bonus to letting the coin make up your mind for you is that sometimes it illuminates feelings you didn't know you had. I tend to flip coins because I really don't care about the options but need to make a choice. Many times, the coin flip tells me I *do* care. I feel my stomach sink as it lands on *heads*; a conclusion of *tails* gives me a thrill of glee. In this way, the penny flip is a win-win; if I truly don't know or care, it can help me get resolution; if I do know or care, it jolts me into a deeper connection with myself. The only drawback is feeling like a weird, obsessive nut flipping coins all the time, but I gave up on appearing "normal" decades ago, and I urge you to follow suit.

JOKER'S WILD

Using a deck of playing cards as a divining oracle is ridiculously simple. The numerical attributions follow that of the Kabbalah's Tree of Life—influential in both the Rider-Waite and Thoth decks—and the suits correspond to basic, pagan elements.

Thereby:

Diamonds = Earth, the realm of the physical, of money, bodies, work, home, health

Spades = Air, the realm of thought, mental activity, communication, conflict, meditation

Clubs = Wands, the realm of passion, creativity, action, good times, war, externalizing

Hearts = Cups, the realm of emotions, feeling, happy and sad tears, moods, internalizing

And:

1 = The origin, new beginning, a fresh start, springtime, turning over a new leaf, new you

2 = Moving from idea to action, just doing it, making the move, daring to strike out, risk

3 = Initial responses and reactions, early success or heartache, seeing if you can trust yourself

4 = Stability, gaining ground, a plan has legs, rest, conservative moves, taking time out

5 = Challenge, fear, worry, disappointment, conflict, frustration, defeat, wiping out, *#fail*

6 = Beauty, success, victory, a big win, sunlight shining on you, everything coming together

7 = Emotionality, lack of control, overthinking, bad coping skills, tears, something isn't working

8 = Math and rationality, making painful decisions, overthinking/spinning out, building systems

9 = The moon, the unknown, grace, fear, letting go, floating, emotional depth, trust, nightmares

10 = Fulfillment, the end of the line, triumph, rewards, stagnation, what's next, celebration

You see that by using this little list, a playing card reading is quite simple. A five of diamonds essentially corresponds to five of disks or pentacles, meaning an upset in someone's material world: money scarcity or fear of poverty, unemployment, unstable work or housing. Two of spades is the same vibe as two of swords: weighing your options, possibly to the extent that you've become paralyzed by overthinking. (Sounds like it's time to flip a coin.)

If, like me, you've got a pretty stuffed game shelf at your home, see if any of them contain cards you can repurpose as divination tools. The Mexican card game Lotería seems like an oracle deck in disguise—the bright images illustrating El Corazón, La Sandía, and El Alacrán seem to be warning that the sweet and juicy love you're courting is bad news! My child has an animal matching card game that does good double-duty as an oracle deck by reading the cultural associations with each critter: a rhino signifies toughness and determination; a turtle slowness and self-protection; a stork represents a gift, or something new on the horizon; a spider suggests a misunderstood artist. Sure, someone else might attribute fear and poison to a spider card, but as the diviner, *you* get to say what the cards you're using signify.

A bag of toys, a bowl of pennies, a stack of playing cards. This all seems to suggest that the business of divination is awfully similar to play, and in my experience, it is—and not just because most major tarot decks on the market are produced by game companies! Tarot *began*, so the legend goes, as the game of Tarrochi; maybe someone recognized the uncanny in the shuffling of the deck, or maybe the game was a protective cover for persecuted pastimes such as fortune-telling. We'll never be sure. Thinking of our lives as a game of Chutes and Ladders, or Towers and Stars, can help us step back and see the big picture of our lives, put a mythological lens on our trials, and help us connect to an ancestry of humans who have suffered and triumphed similarly and used divinatory tools to help them know themselves a little better.

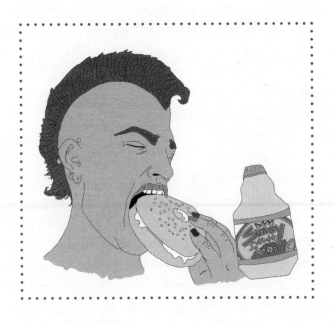

Kitchen Witchery
and Mystical Snacktivism

Growing up with regular meals of Hamburger Helper, Kraft Mac & Cheese, cans of Chef Boyardee, and other packaged edibles, I can't say I had any clue about the potential magic of food. There was a hint, though, during holidays, where boxes and cans were ignored, and actual whole foods were brought in for the feast. Enormous turkeys that had to be ritually cooked overnight. The decorative red glass basket heaped with fruits like a cornucopia, tangerines and grapes and apples tumbling from it like a still life. Root vegetables peeled and boiled and roasted. Even the snacks took on a new, intriguing form: stalks of celery, their canals flooded with cream cheese and dotted with raisins. Sort of gross,

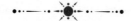

actually, but it was such a *creation*, the novelty got me through a stalk or two.

Even when I returned to taking magic more seriously, in my twenties, I was much too feral to consider how food might be a tool for my practice. A wild alcoholic who was living for the queer nightlife of 1990s San Francisco, I'd sleep late, then stumble to the bagel shop for a salt-studded roll and wash it down with an orange juice. My hangover would dissipate, *as if by magic!* And maybe it was. Those delicious chunks of salt were helping me rehydrate, replenishing what my body lost to chemicals the night before. The magnesium and vitamins I'd tossed into the wind when I was three sheets to it flooded my body as I guzzled the fresh juice. *It's like drinking the sun*, I would think, always, as the flavor jolted my taste buds awake. And like the old alchemists said, "As above, so below." While my breakfast was busy healing my body, my spirit was perking up as well. Salt, any basic witch knows, is a top-notch purifying agent. I'd long been making spray bottles of salty water and hosing down the corners of the room in my punk house, hoping to melt any yucky spirits festering in the corners (a psychic friend had once told me she'd seen *bad energy bats* flapping on my ceiling, and I had become concerned about the metaphysical entities getting tangled in my metaphorical hair). Perhaps the crystals were helping to dislodge any malevolent vibes I'd attracted while on yet another spree, imbibing intoxicants that wore down my aura as much as my immune system. As for the juice, oranges are prized in spellwork for their obvious connection to joy and high spirits; some believe they are connected to the nurturing, femme spirit of our very planet, and others say they carry the vibes of the celestial beings known as angels. They are also very potent in love magic, which is perhaps why I continued to get laid throughout my twenties, even as my addictions rendered me less and less an attractive partner.

Getting sober helped to bring out my latent interest in preparing food. Like most befuddled, newly undrunk people, I thought saying no to booze and snortables would be a simple matter of detoxing my cravings and carrying on. But really, it was a full-scale reckoning with Adulthood. All those basic life skills normies learn while exiting their teen years and moving through their twenties were totally lost on me. I hadn't paid taxes, gotten my teeth cleaned, learned to handle conflict, or dealt with any of my plentiful *issues* in years, if ever. People enter recovery programs not just to have support when getting plastered suddenly seems like a good idea; they do it to find people to hold their hands while they balance their checkbook and clean a fridge for the first time—people who will assure you that you're not a total loser for feeding yourself a diet of canned corn, SunChips, and burritos for the past decade.

It's good to have these major life-skill-building projects to focus on when you're newly sober, because you find that you now have *a lot* of time on your hands. Money, too. All those hours spent planning for the party, becoming the party, and recovering from the party are now free. And, as most of your friends are still on the party cycle, you likely don't have a lot of people to fill your time with either. You will (I did) watch in a sort of awe as the bank balance that stoked a chronic, low-grade anxiety manages to sort of even out, as you are no longer with-drawing blackout cash from sketchy ATMs and handing it over to strangers on street corners and in bar bathrooms. Finally, when you're newly sober, you're *hungry as fuck*. Your body, ac-customed to diabetic levels of sugar from all the malt liquor and wine coolers (what?!) you were giving it, is in a near-constant craving for sweets. Your (my) body is waking up and demanding nourishment. Also, food triggers dopamine, something it takes a newly sober person over a year to replenish after the havoc wreaked.

Early sobriety is an anxious time, an era when habits that soothe are habits that stick. It's also, if you're part of a 12-step program, a moment when you are being urged to turn to spir-itual sources for strength and guidance. I found that the ritual of preparing food—the ASMR of rhythmic chopping; the fresh, damp smells of produce; the melancholy gratitude for animal life taken for sustenance—calmed me, and took me into a somewhat heightened space. And my search for a *higher power* switched my on-again, off-again witch practice to ON. It wasn't hard for these two things to align, as both of them were lighting up my spirit and saving my soul.

I began bringing food to my altar. I was aware that this was a vital part of many practices, from the candy offered to Elegua I'd glimpsed in the botánicas where I bought candles to the glossy oranges heaped before shrines I admired while picking up Chinese takeout. Initially directionless, I gravitated intuitively to things that seemed to represent the sweetness of life, abun-dance, and joy. Citrus fruits were obviously to be revered, with their gorgeous smells and energizing tang. Honey was *clearly* sacred, made from the mysterious bodies of bees in service to their queen, much as I positioned myself before my own altar in reverence to some powerful, femme vibe. Actual candy carried a bit of humor as well as sweetness, and it felt right to include something human-made on my altar. I was, after all, a twenty-first-century city witch. I wasn't walking barefoot into an arbor, conversing with tree nymphs as I plucked fruit from the bough. I was walking through trash and graffiti to grab low-quality produce at my corner bodega. *God is everything, or god is nothing*, my sponsor liked to say, and I began to envision a deity as delighted with the uncanny image of a star in the center of a sliced-open apple *and* a colorful pile of Skittles.

As much as I liked to bring elements from the world I occupied—aka trash—onto my altar (I mean, when you see a playing card in the gutter, don't you have to snag it for your magic spot?), I equally loved being part of a human tradition that had long sourced magic from the stuff of the earth itself. It's not hard to learn what magical properties have traditionally been ascribed to fruits and vegetables, and with the help of occult bookstores and the internet I did (and do) get scholarly about it. I learned that walnuts, my favorite nut, were sacred to the planet Jupiter, handy for spells looking to bring about good fortune and jolly times. Discovering that dandelion, a salad green I was working hard to develop a healthy taste for, was sacred to Aquarius, my sign, strengthened my resolve, and had me integrating a chill cup of dandelion tea into my meditative practice—it's said to support the psychic arts! Peppermint has long been linked to the throat chakra, and its inclusion in a ritually prepared salad or beverage can be a powerful part of rituals intending to help with communication, or summoning the courage to speak truthfully. On and on it goes. Raspberries are stellar for love. Sage, so often burned altar-side, can also be eaten or made into a tea; the earthy nature of the herb is helpful for grounding after you've been wounded or shaken. It heals. Thyme supports new beginnings, especially those moments when we feel we're returning to the world after a hard time. Asafoetida, important to Ayurvedic medicine and delicious curries, is good for holding boundaries and keeping yourself safe. Even something as seemingly mundane as wheat has oodles of magical associations, including wealth, which I happen to adore (and yes, wheat spells are curiously gluten-free). As is cinnamon. Do I smell a cake? Add some vanilla, which amplifies desire, and maybe some apples, which promote success. Actually, let's do this.

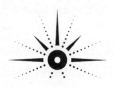

AN ALL-PURPOSE APPLE CAKE
for *Isobel Gowdie*

Isobel Gowdie was an accused witch who died in Scotland in
the late 1600s, one of the last women to be murdered there for
witchcraft, a self-proclaimed *Witch Queen*. Her confessions—
surely given under unbearable torture—are nonetheless the
most detailed, even poetic, account of a woman seduced into
the dark arts that exist. Scholars have tried to explain how
Isobel conjured such specific vignettes, some suggesting she
was a bard or performer, and others musing on a possible
mental illness, perhaps schizophrenia. We do know that Isobel
stuck to her story, even the most minute of details, each of
the four times she was made to confess—something that has
thinkers throughout history scratching their noggins. Isobel,
whom the Devil himself named Jonet (which has a certain
flair, but Isobel is witchier, IMHO), shared that she frolicked
with the head demon in a coven of 13, making that number
magic for all time. Apparently, she also feasted with the king
and queen of fairyland, traveling to their subterranean world
via cavern, and she also had mad orgies with the other witches.
While it does seem most likely that none of this happened, I
earnestly hope that it did. It sounds like a blast.

Being a Scottish woman, Isobel was certainly aware of the place apples held in folk magic. Bobbing for apples, mostly a kid's Halloween game today, began as a bit of romantic divination in Scotland, wherein the first to be married would be divined by whoever first caught a waterlogged apple with their teeth. For a glimpse of who the future spouse could be, the apple was placed beneath the bed to summon prophetic dreams. A similar Scottish trick is peeling an apple in one long, spiraling peel, then looking over your shoulder for a quick glimpse of your dream love. Do it at midnight for extra clarity. Or maybe just bake this all-purpose cake!

I suggest it for a wealth-success-abundance spell, to be whipped up when you're needing a windfall, looking for work, or just calling in resources. But these ingredients are here to help us out in so many matters that this cake is also excellent for radiating a readiness for love; to bless or make sacred a special moment; to kick off a new habit or project to maintain focus on; to cultivate generosity; to support a healing journey; to bring sharpness to scholarly pursuits; to attract good fortune; to honor the dead; to communicate with spirits; to soothe conflict; to conjure bravery; and, frankly, probably any other thing you'd ever do a ritual for.

YOU'LL NEED:

1¾ cups of whole wheat flour

½ cup of unsalted butter, softened, plus more to glaze

¼ cup caster sugar, plus more to sprinkle

4 apples

1 egg

½ teaspoon of milk

Cinnamon for sprinkling

A round, eight-inch pan, ideally greased, lined with
    parchment, and sprinkled with flour

A grater

A clean surface

1. Find a spot in your kitchen to set up a temporary altar.
   Well, I say temporary, but there is so much magic to
   be made in a kitchen, you might just want to keep it
   there! Light a candle, burn some herbs, offer water and
   something of the earth element (salt should be handy?).
   Do whatever you do to put yourself in a heightened space
   of magic-making, whether that is a moment of meditation,
   saluting the elements, or talking to spirits and ancestors.
2. Set the oven to 425°F.
3. Mix the butter and flour in a bowl, cutting the butter into
   the flour with a pastry blender, or mashing and crumbling
   with your hands (sort of more witchy, no?). The butter
   pieces should be small, about the size of a pea.
4. Bring in the sugar.
5. Peel, then grate, two of the apples. Beat that egg. Add them
   both to the bowl and mix it up.
6. This whole time, you're thinking about the effect you want
   this ritual cake to have.
7. You're daydreaming about your future, visualizing. You're
   speaking out loud your desires.
8. Throw that bit of milk into the mixture, so the dough
   doesn't get too stiff.

9. Dump some flour on your clean surface, tip the dough onto it, and knead it softly, really focusing on your magical intentions.

10. Move the charmed dough into the pan, and press it down to create an even surface.

11. Peel and core the remaining apples. Slice them into thick half-moons. Place them on the dough in an appealing pattern. Traditionally, it is a bit of a spiral, which is magically loaded, but feel free to arrange the slices in any way you feel inspired, especially as it pertains to your spell.

12. Melt that extra butter—a tablespoon or two should do it—and brush it over your creation.

13. Sprinkle it with cinnamon and sugar.

14. Bake it in the oven for half an hour.

15. Let the eating of it be part of the ritual, too, whether you enjoy it alone at your altar, in a celebratory group, or with a cutie you're hoping to charm.

SOME NOTES

ON INGREDIENTS: Please splurge for the best ingredients you're able to for this recipe. Not only will it taste better, but animal products from well-cared-for animals and products made by well-compensated humans have better vibes. If you'd like to forgo the animal products altogether, just use plant products. A gluten-free version can be made with almond flour, giving you the magical, abundance-supporting energy of almonds.

ON USING THIS CAKE TO CHARM A CUTIE: I know some
people believe love spells are nonconsensual magical practices.
I will never forget the flyer I glimpsed in a dormitory at
Reed College, where I was teaching at a writing festival. LOVE
SPELLS ARE NOT CONSENSUAL, on hot-pink paper, a classic
love potion illustration with a line through it. While No always
means motherfucking NO, I have my own thoughts about love
spells. When they are done to encourage connection or attract
attention, I think they're swell. When they are done with the
aim of changing someone's mind—like, someone already said no
to you, dumped you, etc.—well, they're creepy. Don't do it.
If you do, it blows up in your face, which is why I ultimately
believe love spells are pretty low stakes. They're not going to
turn someone into a drooling, brainwashed prisoner of love. If
you do a love spell for someone who does not want to be with
you, you're going to see the results pretty fast, in the form of
things going haywire and an abundance of problems. Proceed
accordingly.

ROAD OPENER CHILI

Chili powder is a great tool for unblocking, whether you feel you've been low-key hexed, or if that frustrating call is coming from inside the house. Great for busting out, breaking through, taking a risk, going for it, casting off the bad vibes—yours or someone else's.

YOU'LL NEED:

    2 tablespoons olive oil (Splurge for California if you can; it's the only way to know for sure you're getting actual olive oil and not some sort of unwanted blend)

    1 onion, diced

    4 cloves of garlic, minced

    2 large carrots, chopped

    1 can of kidney beans, drained and rinsed

    1 can of cannellini beans, drained and rinsed

    2 cans of fire-roasted tomatoes

    2 cups of veggie broth

    1 tablespoon chili powder

    2 bay leaves

    1 cup cashews

    Salt and pepper to taste

1. From the moment you gather your ingredients or take a knife to that onion, you are in the ritual. So, be ritualistic. Sing, or dance, or be meditative. Think about or speak aloud what it is you want. Put it into the food you are preparing.

2. In a good, fat-bottomed pot, sauté the onion in olive oil on medium heat for five minutes. Add the garlic, and sauté for an additional minute. Stir these guys around so they don't burn.

3. Add the carrots and sauté for another 10 minutes.

4. Invite the beans to the party, and the tomatoes and broth. Give extra care sprinkling the chili powder, as it is the energetic star of the spell. Bay leaves are also known for bringing victory, so be thoughtful when adding them to the pot as well.

5. Bring to a boil, then reduce to a simmer, keeping it there for twenty minutes to as long as an hour. What will you do during this time? I suggest staying in the ritual of it all. If you have a backyard, go sit on some grass. Meditate. Do a yoga nidra, a deeply relaxing, lengthy meditation that puts your body into a magical, resonant state. Set up an altar. Read your cards, or a spiritual book.

6. About ten minutes before you plan to remove the chili from the stove, toss in the cashews. Pluck out the bay leaves before eating. Eat thoughtfully, meditatively, with intention.

This recipe was inspired by the cashew chili I would eat as a goth teen witch at the Trident Booksellers & Café in Boston.

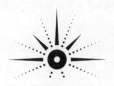

ROSE-COLORED GLASSES LEMONADE

Rosewater is lovely for elevating optimism, and for keeping spirits up during a delay or while in a slump. Add a shot to the likewise sunny elements of lemon, water, and sugar and you've got yourself an elixir to support your summoning of better times.

YOU'LL NEED:

6 cups of water

²/₃ cup of fresh-squeezed lemon juice, from about four big lemons

¼ teaspoon sea salt

1 tablespoon rosewater

1 cup cane sugar

To make this yummy, elevated beverage, simply mix the ingredients and chill, and/or serve over ice.

But do let the ritual of its creation overtake you. Let music or movement be part of it, and do be sure to say aloud and/or meditate upon your desire while mixing.

Sip while visualizing the outcome you'd like to bring into your life, or whatever it is you'd like to manifest.

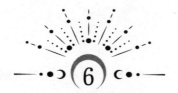

Familiarize Yourself

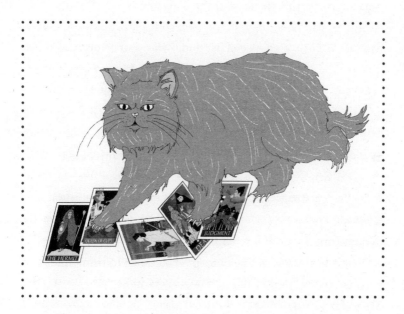

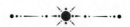

It's a summer day in 2017 and I and my child are at CatCon, a conference for the cat-obsessed. We weren't particularly cat-obsessed—not yet, anyway. We were there as guests of the Con's esteemed featured creature, the famous polydactyl perma-kitten, Lil Bub. I'd become friends with Mike Bridavsky, the man who care-took Lil Bub, who had become internet-famous for her lolling tongue, diminutive stature, and incredible story. Born with a host of genetic anomalies that gave her an otherworldly adorableness and a need for special care, it was a miracle that the feral kitten had survived at all, but as the Universe can be a magical and generous place, Bub found her way to Mike, a very nice artist dude who swiftly organized his life around her care. When his Lil Bub posts went viral, Mike used the attention to snag for her some cutting-edge technology that prolonged her life and relieved her pain (Bub also had her unique genetic makeup sequenced). Using her fame, Mike helped raise over a million dollars for special-needs pets with the ASPCA. As a witch, I'd long known of familiars, animals who have a special, mystical match with a human—they can enhance each other's energies and add sparkle and oomph to magical workings. Mike and Bub seemed like the most fantastic example of the magic humans and animals can make together.

Of course, familiar lore wasn't always so sweet. During the dark days, when superstitions ruled and people suspected of witchcraft were subject to atrocities, the relationships between magical animals and magical people were seen as diabolical. The animals were believed to be demons in disguise, and ate not Kibbles 'N Bits but subsisted on blood from their witch's body. Medieval witch accusers would search for secret breasts on a supposed witch's body, naming moles and skin tags as the spots that fed the beast. Today, people who dabble in paganesque practices (or embrace them fully, or follow a tradition) have reclaimed the idea of a familiar. Witchy folk have a heightened intuition for life energy, and the powerful vibes of the animal kingdom are forever fascinating, both humbling and inspiring. In short, we're pet people.

Historically, though I love animals in theory, I've often found caring for myself to be hard enough. As a kid, I enjoyed the brief life of a lemon-lime parakeet named Petey, who once tweeted us awake when my mom had forgotten to set the alarm clock. That we arrived on time to school was testament to Petey looking out for us, and all the proof I needed that we were connected. As a teenager, sick of my mom blowing off my pleas for a cat, I simply brought home a stray a friend's mom had found at her factory job. I plopped the fluffy black bundle on the kitchen table, and watched my mom fall in love as she fluffily hopped about. The cat was called Nikki, then Jezebel, and then Valor, as I changed her names in accordance with my favorite band at the time.

As an adult, I enjoyed other people's animals. I was an alcoholic, a writer prone to late nights and road trips. The thought of slowing down and acquiring enough stability to tend to a pet felt intimidating, and undesirable. Still, I longed for a special connection with an animal, a creature without language, whom

I would have to rely on intuition to communicate with, growing closer as we studied one another's energies and movements, our friendship taking shape in an uncommon, post/prelingual space. I imagined that animal would somehow just come into my life, unexpected and preordained. Instinctively, we'd know we belonged to each other. What I was hungry for wasn't a pet. It was a familiar.

That day, at CatCon, we left with a kitten. A gray tabby with pronounced, jungly stripes and bat-like ears she hadn't quite grown into, she had a remarkably wild look and a sweet, shy disposition. My son, not quite three, named her Ellie, after the pink elephant in the kid's TV show *Pocoyo*, his current obsession. I adored Ellie, was grateful for the cuteness and whimsy she brought into our house, but it was my then-spouse she chose to snuggle up on each evening, and then lick awake come dawn. She wasn't my familiar.

What makes an animal level up to the bonded witchy person/familiar relationship, anyway? Historically, a witch's familiar wasn't believed to be an animal per se; it was more of an imp or a demon that had taken on the form of an innocuous, common creature to help and support the witch's sinister undertakings. Some beliefs claimed the familiar to be the witch's doppelgänger or alter ego——her self, basically, but able to slip into your home like a mouse, or eat your sheep as a wild dog.

My own feeling about familiars——and, I believe, the common conception of them——is that they are *not* imps or demons or slivers of our own astral-projected spirits. They are themselves, animals, and full of animal magic and personality we love and honor. Because animals seem so at one with their instincts and essence, they can lend that energy to their caretakers and help oomph up the vibrations of our efforts. Will every pet bring that certain energy to the room? Nope. Then, how do you know if your pet is also your familiar? Well, it sounds like a bit of a cop-out, but, when you know, you know. There is an energy, a connection that is stronger, deeper somehow, than the bond you may share with other creatures. Maybe they like to come around when you are engaged in your spiritual practice, entering the room once candles are lit, curling up on your lap when you meditate, or twining around your limbs as you attempt some yoga. I have a friend whose small dog is her faithful companion, a friend she brings with her literally everywhere. But it is her tortoise, a newer relationship, that bolts for her altar whenever she's out of her environment, clambering onto a stack of tarot cards. I got to tortoise-sit this very same reptile for a spell, and, while in a meeting with a publisher about a novel I'd written, the tortoise stationed herself directly under my chair. The publisher bought my novel. This little guy has big familiar energy. But, though I appreciate his goodwill and generosity, he's not *my* familiar.

Six years ago, it was the morning of my child's third birthday, which we were holding in a park. He'd decided upon a rainbow theme, and so we'd gotten a rainbow-frosted cake and plates and a giant cardboard rainbow to dangle from the trees. Sporting a rainbow-striped terrycloth headband and matching wristbands, he jumped up and down by the front door with his three-year-old cousin, antsy to get on with it. The door was hung with bags of snacks and decorations, and as I pulled it open, a cat ran in! Well, he didn't run. He sort of sauntered. He swaggered. He had, even in his bedraggled state—careworn and dirty, a little too bony, possibly harboring some stowaway fleas—a sort of *joie de vivre*. We made way for him to enter, a black-and-white tuxedo cat, his markings like that of a cow. With his pointy black ears and black fur running mask-like over his yellow eyes, he looked not unlike Batman.

Loaded down with supplies, I couldn't stop him, and I watched with alarm as my son, a graceless toddler, dove for the cat and lifted him up awkwardly. "Don't!" I yelled. "Stop! Put him down!" But my child did not put him down, only giggled and guffawed as he worked to balance the cat's slinky weight. He passed the furry beast to his cousin, an avowed cat lover, who also flung the feline around clumsily, in the boorish manner of toddlers everywhere. "Stop!" I continued to crow. "Don't!" But the kids didn't care, and neither, remarkably, did the cat. I waited for a claw to the face, a startling hiss, at the very least a meow of complaint. But the cat did nothing. Released from the tiny ogres, he slunk deeper into our home. He spied Ellie's new-fangled, modern cat bed that did an okay job of not looking like the ugly piece of cat furniture it was, and slid into its cavernous cubby. He gazed at us coolly, closed his eyes, and went to sleep.

One of my favorite pictures of my son is from later that day. His hair grimy, spiky with sweat and dirt, his face ruddy from running and screaming his way through his party, he is sprawled in my bed, still in his rainbow attire. And sprawled along the length of him, skin-to-fur, is Birthday Rainbow, the name my son gave the cat when I agreed that we could keep him. My agreement, incidentally, felt ridiculous; I didn't feel I had any say in the matter. Birthday Rainbow walked into the house, demonstrated his epically chill demeanor by letting the toddlers manhandle him, made fast friends with Ellie, and called us home. The decision was all his.

I think that Birthday Rainbow is my familiar, a wild, freedom-loving cat who jibes with the type of care and love I have for a pet. Sober now, and stable, I can get him his two squares, scoop his litter, and squirt him with flea meds every month. I love taking care of him, how he climbs into my lap while I'm meditating, the annoying way he marches across the tarot reading spread out on the floor. And though I deeply feel that he is mine, and I am his, I don't believe that I *own* Birthday Rainbow. He's not *my* cat. He's his own cat, entitled to the life he desires, which is why I'm okay with opening the door all day and all night to let him come and go as he pleases. Mostly he lounges on the porch, but occasionally he has followed us on walks around the block, and once he came home with a note tucked into his collar, written by another family who occasionally feeds and pets him. More than once I've spotted his picture on community message boards online, and had to assure the concerned citizens that yes, he has a home, is loved and cared for, and I do know there are coyotes, not to mention cars, out there in the big world; there are raccoons and dogs and people up to no good, but this is his world, Birthday

Rainbow's, and he wants to be a part of it. I understand. I've always wanted to be a part of the big, bad world, too, dangers be damned. Sometimes he doesn't come home for a day, maybe even two, and my heart plops down a level and rolls around in my stomach. Is this it? Did Birthday's clock get punched? I get a taste of the real grief that awaits me when the inevitable occurs. But it hasn't occurred yet. Inevitably, I see him jump up into the kitchen window and start meowing into the glass, yelling at me to let him in.

Me and Birthday haven't always had it easy. During one dark era, when my home was plagued with illness and cat pee, I tried to rehome him. It shocks me now to think of it, and I feel shame, too, and then I realize I've fallen out of touch with how scared and desperate I'd felt. I'm glad that no one wanted him. I've apologized and made him promises I'm prepared to keep. He'll still up and piss all over my kid's stuffed animals every now and then, for no apparent reason, but there's enzyme spray and vinegar and the unconditional love I have for him in my heart, and we get through it. I do believe he is my familiar; I see myself in his unfussy, vagabond vibe, and I think he recognizes in me a similar scent. He has killed one of my child's pet hamsters and maimed another, and all the birds and lizards of the neighborhood fear his yellow eyes. I know that one day he will fall to the wild fierceness of another beast, and though I will mourn him and miss him, I will respect the way he lived and died, gentle yet untamed, autonomous and loving, not submitting to his nature but reveling in it. A pure and earthy death, a death that makes sense, a death that gives life. Until then, he will curl up on my desk and watch me as I work at my altar, lending, I like to believe, his distinctive essence to the work, as he's lent it to the lives of everyone around him.

MEOW, SATHAN: A SPELL TO CALL A FAMILIAR

Elizabeth Francis, born in England in 1529, had a life as rough as any medieval femme—she was beggar-level broke, her rich boyfriend wouldn't marry her (then he went broke, and died), and when she finally did get married it was to a tumultuous brute. Their one baby died at six months. She was also the first person brought to trial under the Witchcraft Act of 1562, which applied a death sentence to witches who used magic to murder.

Although we can never know for sure, it's pretty safe to assume many of the outlandish accusations hurled against Francis—which she admitted to under the horrors of torture—were hogwash, so allow me to pick and choose what I would like to believe. Her witchy grandmother had made her a witch at the age of twelve, gifting her a white spotted cat named Sathan. History insists that Sathan spoke to Francis in a "strange, hollow voice," which is thrilling to imagine. Like all medieval familiars, Sathan subsisted on blood, but only just a drop, from Francis's finger, mixed into his regular meal of milk and bread. For this, Sathan swore to "fulfill her needs," providing sheep, mostly.

Elizabeth Francis was tried a whopping three times before being found guilty of witchcraft; the third trial contained testimony that Francis was seen feeding bread to a shaggy ghost dog she then sicced on a woman who was being stingy with her yeast. Medieval problems! The yeast hoarder testified that the ghost dog had given her a terrible pain in the head.

In memory of Elizabeth Francis, who surely did love her cat and who suffered so tragically from the idiocy of her place and time, I offer a spell to bring to you your own loyal Sathan or shaggy dog, or pigeon or gecko or whatever type of animal you long to have a familiar relationship with into your life.

This spell works best on a full moon, as animals are so responsive to the fullness of our satellite (as are we, animals also!). You are looking to connect with the energy of your special beast. Think about the element most likely associated with the animal you wish to friend. Mammals and land animals are earth, fish and turtles are water, winged animals are air. Reptiles can take fire, as they need warmth (and there's a myth that the salamander can exist within fire). Make sure the element has pride of place on your altar or magical space— you might have a crystal or a big pile of dirt, and maybe a plant, for earth; a goblet of water for water; a feather for air; a candle for fire. If you have a figurine that represents your animal, use it. The most important energy between you and your familiar will be love, so bring in some flowers known for that: jasmine, roses, poppies, hibiscus, lilacs. Place a piece of bread and a small bowl of milk, plant or animal, on your altar. Sit before your altar and daydream about your familiar. Imagine what they look like, where they might be. Call out to them from your heart and from your mind. Have a whole conversation with them inside your head. When you feel that you've expressed yourself to your familiar, spend some time visualizing being with your familiar, either in this world, in the mundane ways you expect to hang out, or in some sort of fantasy magic-land doing wild, witchy things. Or both!

When you're done with your spell, take the milk and bread and leave it someplace outside for an animal. Whatever eats it probably isn't your familiar. But who knows? Racoons are cute! It's but an offering to the animal world. Now, go about finding your familiar, carrying the feeling of the ritual inside your heart.

BONDING WITH YOUR FAMILIAR

Try deepening your connection to your familiar by setting up a special altar for them. Using the elemental associations I mentioned above, plus any other materials that represent them—a shed whisker or feather, a toy, etc.—light a candle (shades of blue and purple are best) and meditate for a bit about the type of energetic exchange you want to have with your familiar. Do you want a stronger vibe, a tighter frequency? Do you want to get wild and run around? Would you like them to visit you in your dreams? When you've established what you'd like, come out of meditation and go to them. Tell them what you would like. If you are trying to establish a stronger psychic bond, get close and cuddly. Play gently. Make good eye contact and speak to them. If you want their wildness, rev them up and feel the charged exchange. This is primarily energy work, difficult to prescribe exactly, but the combination of ritual and intentional presence and time will get you the depth you're desiring.

TO LET GO OF A LOST FAMILIAR

One of the biggest lessons our animal friends teach us is the fleetingness of life. There is no saying hello to a familiar without saying an eventual goodbye. When you are ready to let go of your beloved familiar, bring to your altar the biggest chunk of rose quartz you can get your hands on. Rose quartz is love, unconditional love, the sort of love you and your familiar shared, and the kind your heart surely needs right now. Burn fragrant herbs to purify you and your space and help move energy along. Use an iron cauldron or fireproof bowl. Begin by sitting in the smoke with the rose quartz, meditating on the love you have for your familiar. Let the tears come. Feel all your feelings, whatever they are, but be sure to add gratitude to the mix. Think about all the ways you are grateful to your familiar, and for your time together. Come out of your meditation, and write down your thoughts on paper. Everything you got from your pet, everything they offered you. At your cauldron or fireproof bowl, express your gratitude out loud to your familiar's spirit. Thank them. Tell them it is okay to move on to their next adventure. Assure them you will be okay—and know that you truly will be. Burn the paper in the bowl, offering the smoke and the fire as more gratitude and love. Your beloved familiar has moved on, but you are still here on Earth, an animal among animals. When the fires have gone out, bring your rose quartz to bed with you, and sleep with it near your pillow until you have a significant dream of an animal. Be sure to write the dream down. Was it your familiar? Is it the energy of a future animal companion? Or was it you, expressing something about your relationship to your familiar's memory, or the magic of the animal kingdom more broadly?

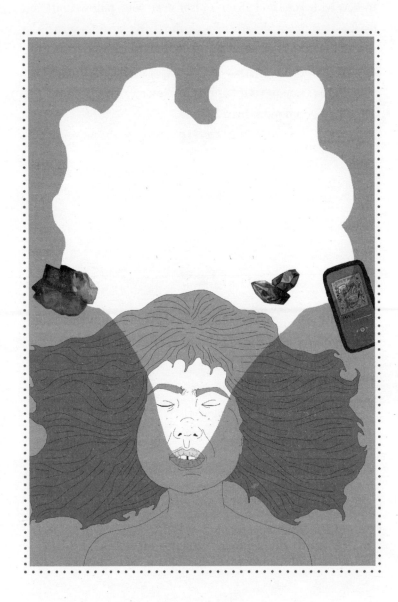

Catch Your Breath

I always knew that breathing was cool. Sort of. As an Aquarius, I've always had a rough time connecting with my body. Well, *rough* makes it sound like there was an effort, some struggle. There wasn't. There was just, like, nothing. Privileged with good physical health, I just didn't think that much about my flesh and bones. It was a vehicle for my brain, I figured, and I enjoyed flooding it with sensation via sex and drugs, but that was about it. In my twenties and into my thirties, when folks around me were getting sweaty at yoga classes and talking about how *grounding* it was, I listened with mild curiosity; the mystical element sounded cool but I didn't like *sports*. The sports I was around tended to be the occasional butch friend tearing their ACL playing rugby, or a girlfriend who spent her Saturday mornings playing soccer in a part of the

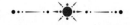

city I'd never been to. Exotic! But not for me. I'd heard about *breathwork*, or that you could legit get high from manipulating your breath, but it seemed like the sad sort of consolation sober people gave themselves—*I don't need to party, I'm high on breath!* I'd get high on snortables like a normal person, thank you very much, and as for breathing, it was mainly for smoking.

Little did I know that breathing, this thing we do on autopilot, is actually a magic practice that is *right under our nose*. There are truly ancient Asian practices that have long understood that our breath, should we become conscious and deliberate about it, can be a way for us to deepen our connection with the divine, both inside and outside of our selves. In the United States, breathing, via meditation and yoga, appears to have been absorbed by general wellness culture, a realm that too often seems to be about getting ourselves in top form so that we may better perform our social roles as worker, mother, producer—a stealth capitalist enterprise to better ourselves for capitalism.

Trapped as we all are *in* capitalism, magic does interact with this system (a witch has gotta eat too, no?), but the magic I'm interested in provides us with routes to get outside of these and all systems that threaten to rob us of our wonder, liberty, agency, and divine spark. So yeah, I was pretty gobsmacked to learn that something as basic and universal as breathing could catapult me into realms that felt drenched in mysticism and magic.

Let me set the scene. I was sober, not smoking, and a mom to boot. My witch practice had been reclaimed and was fully engaged. I was living on the east side of Los Angeles, where you can't swing a big hat without hitting a breathwork or sound bath session. And I had *still* never done either. But when a mom at my kid's preschool shared that she was hosting a breathwork session as a fundraiser for the school, I signed up, more as an engaged parent than a spiritual seeker.

A word about this preschool. It was a co-op, which meant parents committed to working as teachers and running the school, alongside a handful of paid experts. This kept the cost low, handy for low-income parents, but meant you had to have a lot of free time, hard for low-income parents. My then-spouse and I were in the middle, economically, and made it work. Everyone was required to attend nonviolent parenting workshops, fascinating lectures on the development of the human brain and nervous system, and were taught parenting methods and conflict resolution styles informed by the fritzy, fledgling wiring of our children's psyche. Like me, most of the other parents weren't raised so thoughtfully, and there was much tearful sharing during sessions.

I'd arrived at the school a bit proud of what I had to offer, in particular my tarot reading skills, which I was ready to monetize on the organization's behalf. Come to learn, Los Angeles in the mid-2010s was (still is) *crawling* with witchy moms. I met a mom who'd just returned from an in-depth psychic sleepaway camp at a Hogwarts-like spot in England. Another mom was studying herbalism, soft-launching a business that made organic firewaters and apoptogenic teas. There was a mom who offered guided meditation and visualizations, and another whose specialty was breathwork. As every family was charged with raising

a certain amount of cash for the school, this mom was present-
ing a breathwork session in the back cottage of her home on a
Sunday morning, and I signed up.

I liked this mom. She was a tall white woman, willowy yet
strong, with choppy blond hair often fading out from some color
not found naturally in hair. I liked all the moms at the preschool,
and I was excited for a chance to hang out and be mellow together, away from the kids on a weekend morning. Because that's
what it would be, right? Breathwork? Something like meditation,
sitting and breathing together, maybe with some imagery like a
tree-trunk tail growing out of our spine and into the earth, that
sort of thing. I'd been around the new age block and knew what
to expect.

We gathered, about ten of us, on the top floor of the cottage,
slanted-ceiling attic vibes, cozy. All of us were moms of fairly
young children, and for many of us, like me, it was our first time
having this all-encompassing experience. Our leader, River, lit
candles, as we each found a place to post up with the blankies
and pillows we'd been instructed to bring. Slumber party vibes,
I thought, that experience of being in an all-girl space, with girls
you know from school, familiar in some ways and strangers in
others. I figured I'd maybe fall asleep, what tended to happen if
I allowed my body to relax for more than a couple of minutes.
My child was three; it had been a wild few years.

River had us get comfortable, lying on our backs. She instructed us in the breathing technique, the first sign that this
was not a regular meditation. The breaths were taken in three
steps: an inhale through the nose into the belly, then up into

the chest, and then released through the mouth, all with no pauses—full, deep, and constant. Each breath connected to the next, a track of breath running like a train from our nostrils to our core and back through our mouths. "You might feel tingling sensations in your hands and feet," she prepped us. "Sometimes you feel your upper lip sort of curl up over your gums. And you might cry." Okay, weird, but none of that shit would happen to me. Though getting sober, and having a baby, had surely left me more connected to my body than I'd ever been, I was still, at center, an Aquarian. I believed the subtleties of body magic—breathing, sound, flower essences, acupuncture—would somehow be lost on my system. It's why I'd needed rough sex and hard drugs to feel my earthly form. Something about my nature required a sledgehammer to get rooted.

Could breath be a sledgehammer? Once I got into the rhythm of my breathing—a pattern that felt like a loop, even as it traveled up and down the length of me—I realized I would probably not take a nap after all. It required some effort to keep these breaths coming. Also, there was music, and not the tinkly chimes one tunes out during a massage. It was unexpectedly poppy, and *loud*. I kept at my breathing, in and out, in and out, and began to feel the sort of tingling I'd been warned about, in my hands and feet, in my knees. I breathed into it. *Whoa.* As I worked my breath—hardly work at all, now, but moving on its own propulsive energy, *loop, loop, loop*—the music pummeled me in a new way, getting under my skin. Was I breathing the music? Psychedelic thoughts began to flutter into consciousness. I felt lightheaded, maybe, but I was laying down so it was hard to know. Everything was merging: my breath, the chaos of the music, the wild tangle of it all throbbing inside my chest like a living thing. My upper lip, buffeted by the wind of my breath, did in fact grow dry and begin to climb my gums. I felt it stuck up there, weird, but I ignored it and kept going. This was not *at all* what I thought it would be. This was not a gentle visualization that left me pleasantly spacey; it wasn't Meditation 101 where I fought with drifting thoughts. This was a whole new thing.

River moved about us like a conductor of sorts, placing crystals from a basket near people's feet or crowns. I didn't know she was doing this; I didn't know where she was or what she was doing, but I had a sense of her, as if my third eye was surveying her. In the pause between songs, she would have us repeat an affirmation. "I am whole healing," she prompted us, and I didn't even throw up in my mouth at the thought of speaking such an easy-cheesy statement into the air. *Healing*—which I understand is a *thing*, even, arguably, a thing I have been *involved in* for a couple decades—is also a thing that has had so much new-agey white light barfed upon it that it scarcely means anything to me, anymore. But in that little mom-stuffed room, that day, I felt differently. The psychedelic thoughts—embarrassingly simple sentiments like *Love is all that matters* felt with new, raw power—entered on what felt like an internal arctic wind that blew all the muck inside me into some psychic gutter. I felt it as a gust that cleansed a part of me I hadn't known needed a scrub. *Cleanliness is next to godliness*, I thought, a psychedelic thought, meaning it sounds silly now but had hit me physically, wracking me with an untranslatable truth.

River started another song. Familiar, at first, though I tried not to let it perk up my intellect, that seeking mind that wants to know everything. A different region of my mind had come online, maestro of the psychedelic thought, both ridiculously basic and extremely wise. It was "Do You Realize??" by the Flaming Lips, I realized as the singer began his query. *We're floating in space*—yes, yes, we are, but I knew where this song was going, and that sassy part of my brain cursed, *River, oh, River, you diabolical shaman, you little mystic minx, you're really going to take us out now, aren't you?*

Do you realize / That everyone you know will someday die? Well. I had heard the sniffles, as I breathed through my wonderland, of the women around me managing sinus cavities newly impacted by a crying jag. I hadn't thought too much about it—we were all new-ish moms, more or less, hadn't slept much in the past three or four years, had probably reckoned with postpartum mood swings and certainly had had our hormones tossed into the air like a game of 52-card pickup. In this state, we worked daily to bend feral creatures to our will. None of us were strangers to crying. But now I was crying, too. Because *everyone I knew someday would die.* Me. My partner. *Our baby.* Our child. Impossible. Could happen anytime. Not that there was anything fatal afoot, just, you know, whoever thinks they're on the precipice of a surprise, life-changing tragedy? My breath, till now steady on its track like a car turning corkscrews in the darkness of Space Mountain, became ragged. I slipped off my track. I made a sound, a light sob. I heard similar gasps around me. I imagined, briefly, River leaning against the wall, in the glow of candlelight, smiling a benevolent smile on us, her charges, as we wept and newly confronted that old bugaboo, our mortality. What a witch! The tears slid down the edges of my eyes, streaming into my ears, which felt awful. I moved my hands, to swat and itch—what were these clumsy, thick gadgets? They were weighty and buzzing like a hive full of honey. I let them plop down. I got back into my rhythm. It wasn't hard.

River had us shouting more affirmations. *I accept today. I am at peace. I am love.* At the end, instead of another phrase to sear into our spirit, she had us scream. And we did. A room of women screaming, a room of screaming mothers.

"Take your time coming back to yourself," River began to gently end the session. "Take your time opening your eyes, moving your body." As if we could have done anything else. We were stunned, all of us. Like pill bugs slowly unrolling, we rattled our legs, jazz-handed our wrists, pulled the husk of a lip back over our parched gums. River had given us all paper and pens to record any big thoughts we'd had during our trance. All around me, people were lying on their bellies, scribbling. My mind reeled with what to write. Like a rock whose magic sparkle catches your eye in the ocean, I knew to pull it out would only cause it to dry up and lose its magic. *Why did I bring this rock home with me again?*

The thought that was resonating the hardest, throbbing like a fresh cut, was *clarity*. I had never experienced anything like it. Like a film had been scraped from my mind. I felt a little amped, but also peaceful. Energized. Joyful, in spite of my recent tears, in spite of everyone I know having a death sentence, in spite of my own. I jotted it down as best I could, knowing it probably didn't matter. I probably wouldn't ever look at this piece of paper again. But I would breath like this again. That I knew.

Breathwork has been an off-again, on-again practice for me since that day. I began going to River's group breathwork sessions, breathing in a row of other breathers, welcoming the familiar tingles and tears as I moved into a deeper space. Sometimes I would feel a spinning sensation above my heart—my heart chakra. I feel lucky to occasionally feel these vortexes and their connections to my physical form, whether it is the speedy swirl of a heart chakra as it opens itself to a crush, or the spiral of energy I sometimes feel at the crown of my head as I'm falling asleep. The buzz of my third eye, making me wake up and pay attention with its nearly unbearable tickle. The opening of my heart chakra in breathwork was something I would feel again and again. At the time, my partner and I were on the verge of opening our relationships. I was scared it would go badly; indeed, it arguably would, yet I stand, years later, in my new life, quite happy. As my heart space whorled open, I knew I was meant to walk bravely, openly, into this experience. I would fall in love and get my heart multiply broken. It was, I realized with psychedelic clarity, what my heart was meant to do.

There have been challenging times with breathwork, as well. Connecting with the eternity, the infinity, of *love* during a session, I had to restrain myself from texting numerous exes messages that would have been concerning, if not wholly unwelcome. Consensus reality does not often merge well with mystical states, and I'm grateful I followed the hunch that such offerings of cosmic devotion would only lead to me cleaning up a mess I'd barely be able to explain. I just sat with it. It is a form of meditation, after all. The point is to feel that surge of love, without beginning and without end, and know that I am all caught up in its stream, that I may even be its source. Like all highs—and lows for that matter—its best to hold on lightly, and release.

Another time I was doing breathwork alone, in the room I work and do magic in. I began my home breathwork practice slowly, skittishly—though I had never had a negative experience, it was such an overwhelming one, I liked knowing that River was there, competent and tethered to the earth, in case I needed help grounding. But my home sessions were more or less like the group ones I'd experienced, and I enjoyed making my own playlist—like River, diabolically placing a song with a powerful message, like Yoko Ono and Cat Powers's "Revelations," smack in the middle when I knew I would be most vulnerable to its message. After breathing (in a circle of crystals) in my room, I'd rise, journal, read tarot, and drift downstairs for a snack. For a while this was my regular practice, and I entertained the thought of having a bunch of friends curious about the exercise over to my house, to guide them through it as River had guided me.

Then, Covid hit. And I got divorced, my polyamory path leading me into the terrain best illustrated by the Tower card in the tarot, an arcana that came for me frequently then. One evening, late-ish at night, alone in my giant home, my child spending the week with my now-ex and their now-new-partner, I laid on my floor and entered into the familiar pattern of breath. The tears came swiftly—had they ever gone away? I cried around the clock then, a hot summer of tears that left me dehydrated and subsisting on a diet of popsicles. My breath locked itself into the glowing, familiar loop, and my tears turned to sobs, turned to weeping. I kept going. I recognized this practice as a healing one now, any cringe associations with that word be damned. It was a truth, healing, and I felt it most palpably in this state. But this time, rather than bringing searing clarity, my breaths brought doom. The weight of my grief was too much for me; the stark, psychedelic pain felt like a legendary myth, something that had predated me, a destiny I had finally locked myself into. All was lost. There was no joy, there was no love. There was just *this*, a terrible void, a malevolent abyss. The absence of love, felt on a cataclysmically grand scale.

I stayed in that session longer than I should have. I am someone who always wants *the truth*, no matter how devastating. Inside the heightened experience of breathwork, the truth of my pain became epic, grand enough to obliterate the reality of love I'd so often felt before. *That was a lie*, my grief told me. *Only this is real.* It was unbearable to face, but I made myself engage with it, until I didn't. I broke the glowing loop of breath and shook myself out of the physical trance. I crawled into child's pose and wept and wept. The knowledge of a place without love, a psychic realm of sorts, was in me now, and though it seemed intolerable, I tolerated it, accepted it. It was a truth. Was it the only truth? Did the pain of my shadow revelation necessarily obliterate the sunnier epiphanies breathwork had brought? It took me a little while to figure it out, and I could probably write a book solely about that journey, how part of me still feels like I'm on it every day. Like a flash of bad lightning, my grief came down and made a negative out of everything good in this realm. I don't regret this powerful vision. I stayed away from breathwork for a while, until I felt my grief relocate itself in my psyche, and relocate again. Like love, it never goes away. It flavors my breathwork now, which has become about taking in the unfathomable everythingness of life, holding it in this particular way that accents the mystery of it, its essential mystical nature. My breathwork recommendation comes with warnings now. Like any psychedelic, it might emphasize your baseline state. If you're in a bad place, it might take you deeper into that bad chamber. Sometimes that is healing; sometimes it's just too much. You get to decide your limits. No one gets an award for being a hero here; if you feel your pain has a worth to it, a purge, a comfort, then stay—but if it is just wigging you the fuck out and you want to bolt, please do. A partner whose anxiety often manifested through breath found themselves unable to go very deep into the practice without summoning panic; another time, I was leading a group session as part of a writing workshop, and one student had to shake herself out of it and leave the room, as the intensity did not feel welcoming.

Breathwork engages our consciousness and our psyche. Our breath delivers oxygen to our entire physical form, and so all of our body is impacted by this work. It is intense in its gifts and, I've learned, in its harder lessons. If you seek to know this practice, I encourage you to find a group workshop helmed by an instructor; there are many of these available, and many offered online as well as in person. Know yourself, your tendency toward anxiety or breathing issues. This doesn't necessarily block you from this practice—I have a generalized anxiety disorder diagnosis, and I was able to practice happily for months before having my experience impacted by life circumstance. But it is good to know that you bring your whole self into this magical practice, and any aspect of you could arise.

BASIC BREATHWORK

To prep, find a spot where you will be comfortable and undisturbed, a place that has nice-to-neutral vibes. I've done breathwork in beds, but I actually prefer the floor—you want it to feel different than going to sleep. You can lie on the floor upon a yoga mat, or blankets; have a blanket handy to cover you as well, since sometimes folks get cold during this practice. I like to activate my altar smoke and candles, and to select special crystals to bring into the ritual. I have made circles of stones and lain within them, and I have also placed stones on or near my chakras—they'll roll off sometimes, but it's okay. I do *not* recommend holding crystals in your hands. I once did this, only to find that my hands sort of crumpled up into strange claws *around* the stones, and it took a bit to come out of the trance and for my hands to relax and release them. It didn't feel great!

Put a playlist together. It might seem like slow-tempo,

mystical tunes are the way to go, but as I experienced in my class with River, pop songs can also become quite profound under the spell of breathwork; psychedelic experiences are great for transforming the simplest sentiments into something deeply profound. Upbeat songs with positive messages are excellent, as are soulful songs of any genre. One old playlist I still have on my phone starts with Cramps's rockabilly ode to the vagina, "Hot Pearl Snatch"; segues into the gorgeous and mystical "Dazzle" by Siouxsie and the Banshees; dips into The Smiths's rebellious ode to love, "Sheila Take a Bow"; roars into Mötley Crüe's "Shout at the Devil" (okay, a bit on the nose); and ends with the empowering "50ft Queenie," by PJ Harvey. This is what my psyche responds to. Make your list one that will captivate your own subconscious. And yes, you only need five songs.

Play the music as loud as you can. If you're using a phone, as I do, place it by the crown of your head, so it is close and the sound is balanced. Begin breathing—deep breath through the nose, taken all the way into your belly, then into your chest, then released through your mouth, only to be *immediately* inhaled through your nose again. Continue this, observing the changes you experience in your body and mind, the way you react to the music you've selected. If it feels like too much at any time, cease breathing in such a way. Just breathe normally, move your body, sit up. Get yourself something to eat or a glass of water. If it feels safe and interesting, stay in it. I like to keep a journal and tarot cards handy; the state of increased profundity breathwork offers is great for tarot. I also like to do some gentle yoga to get back into my body, and then have a snack.

|||||||||||||||||||||||||||||||||||||||||||||||||||||||||||||||||||

FAIRY BREATHS FOR BIDDY EARLY

|||||||||||||||||||||||||||||||||||||||||||||||||||||||||||||||||||

U sing the basic breathwork technique detailed above, it is possible to set certain intentions before entering the breath trance and source specific information for your psyche. This ritual is in honor of Biddy Early, an Irish fairy-doctor who died in the late 1800s. Biddy was known throughout her region for being a powerful healer, and she gave all credit to her gifts to the fairy folk, who she communed with and who she said taught her how to heal with herbs and to divine the future. The fairies had gifted Biddy with a special blue bottle, via her son, who also had occult gifts, assuring him that Biddy would know how to use it. The lore goes that the bottle was prone to filling with a vapor, and that Biddy would scry it before helping a seeker. If the mist did not appear, she would know that she was unable to cure the person, and would decline to work with them. After her death in 1874, the magic bottle was flung into her local Loch Kilgarron, where it would sink to the bottom, never to be utilized again.

In this breathwork ritual, the intention is to make contact with the "good people," another name for the fairy folk of Biddy's place and time, who were understood to be among them. Now, there is a yet-to-be-proven (or unproven) theory that breathwork releases the psychedelic chemical DMT (dimethyltryptamine). You might have heard of DMT as a main component of ayahuasca. Psychonauts report visions of otherworldly entities when taking

ayahuasca. Mystical ethnobotanist Terence McKenna spoke of
encountering "self-transforming elf machines" while on a DMT
journey. Others have reported meeting aliens, cats, praying
mantids, and other creatures, all of them vibing benevolent,
intelligent vibes.

DMT is found in our pineal gland—yes, the physical site
of our mystical third eye. A sad-sounding study done on mice
(just sad, right?) concluded that, when under stress, the mice's
pineal glands secreted DMT, and, so goes the theory, the stress
that breathwork temporarily puts upon our body may make our
own brains squirt out some of this groovy stuff, which would
account for why the experience is so darn psychedelic.

Terence McKenna's elves, Biddy Early's fairies—could they
be the same? To attempt to make contact with these ethereal
beings, I did a shout-out to Biddy herself, asking for her attention and care from the spirit realm. I burned a blue candle on
my altar alongside water and smoke. If you have a blue bottle,
by all means fill it with water and smoke, if you can, and offer
it to the Irish witch. Ask her to be with you as you take this
journey, and to connect you with the beings on the other side
of this reality. Then, begin your breathwork.

Perhaps the hardest part is keeping your mind open to messages and visions from these creatures. As with most things
psychic, I find it hard to simply trust myself. Am I getting a
message, or am I making shit up? Multiple conversations with
psychics who have *less* imposter syndrome than I do assure me
it's all one and the same. When we source for otherworldly
communication, it's going to come through the same channels

as our imagination. You have to take a massive, fool-sized leap, and believe that what you see and hear is sacred in origin, and has a message for you.

For this breathwork session, classical music might be best, as it is less likely to trigger specific mental activity the way language does. Be sure to journal right after leaving your trance. Unlike the gibberish I scratched out following my first breathwork experience, you might be dictating clues to a parallel universe that has long existed alongside humanity, showing up in our myths and legends.

And be sure to thank Biddy when you're through.

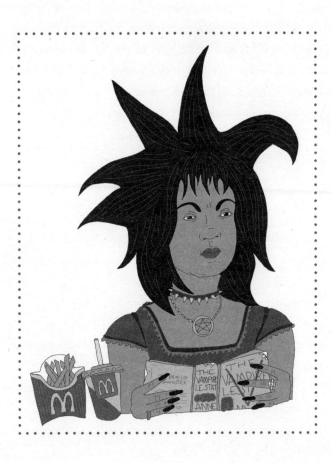

Hex Marks the Spot

F or as long as the world has known of them, witches have
been synonymous with hexes—the ability to summon
a personal, mystical power to do harm. Perhaps that's
the reason why some modern witches take a stand against
the practice—it's a drag to be defined by one single element of
witchery, especially a "negative" one. Such ignorance surely
fed ancient suspicion and hatred of witches, and it makes sense
to want to be known as the holistic, good-vibes witch you
probably are. Sometimes it seems like the trend against hexing is part of a larger rebranding scheme, spinning witches as
kinder and gentler.

But I've never been one for respectability politics.

I'm not alone in such a rebellious stance. Just as there
are witches who give hexing a hard no, there are many who

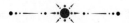

affirm the destructive aspects of magic as a sacred aspect of the Goddexx, she with the power to destroy as well as create. To ignore the so-called shadow side of magic—the will to break, to wreak havoc, to stunt or sicken or bind—does seem to rob us of a pantheon of global dark goddesses, deities whose wrath, much like our own, so often comes from understandable causes. There is much pain in the world, much injustice, and we experience the gamut of it, everything from a romantic affair gone unfairly sour to belonging to a people being targeted with extreme violence and oppression. In the face of it all, renouncing hexing can seem like shortsighted, ridiculous virtue signaling.

I cast my first hex when I was a teenager, just at the very start of my practice. I certainly wasn't calling myself a witch, not yet, and had probably only burned some intentional incense in my bedroom at that point. I had a bundle I'd bought on a day trip to Salem, labeled *For Courage.* I needed it. The way I liked to look—big, teased hair, thrift store dresses, clown-white pancake makeup and religious jewelry—as I mentioned before, it wasn't regarded kindly in my hometown of Chelsea, Massachusetts, circa 1986. I got a lot of shit, most of it mouthy, but I'd also experienced the not-infrequent projectiles tossed from speeding cars, and so many threats of an ass-kicking it sort of felt like it had already happened. Sometimes it was hard to leave the house knowing that people were going to say mean, foreboding things to me, but I *loved* how I looked, and I also knew these people were fucking assholes. I teased my box-black hair a little higher and applied a fresh coat of the Elvira-brand

Halloween-season black lipstick I wore year-round, and got on with my life.

One afternoon, after the school bus from my dreary regional vocational high school in the sticks had burped me out, I realized I'd left my keys at home and was locked out. I knew my mom would be off her nursing shift at the Soldiers' Home in an hour or so, and I decided to wait it out at the McDonald's on my corner. It was close, it was cheap; I bought a bag of fries and huddled in a booth with my paperback copy of *The Vampire Lestat*, exploded-looking with ragged pages because I'd been reading it on a constant loop for some time. I was able to focus on a story I loved so intensely that it blocked out the world around me—the television chaos at home, the cruel chatter at school, the insults hurled at me on public transit. But this time, the jeering penetrated my little bubble of New Orleans vampiric romance. I was being ogled, and taunted. By *children*.

I looked around the "restaurant" to see where the parents of this group of young—ten, twelve-year-old—ruffians were, so I could lodge a complaint about their offspring. Not that that was a guaranteed font of justice—these little jerks tended to learn their xenophobia at home, and a parent was as likely to cosign my harassment as put an end to it. But no matter, there weren't any parents around. This was a pack of feral, free-range Chelsea children.

My direct gaze, my *scowl*, did nothing but give them a better look at my elaborate makeup, prompting more snorts and insults. "Are you a Satanist?" one kid ribbed, as it was the 1980s and the "satanic panic" was afoot. But in that moment, I realized, yes, yes, *of course* I was a Satanist. I was so bothered that this gaggle of *children* wasn't afraid to mess with me, a *teenager*, a potentially *Satanic* teenager, that inspiration struck.

I was wearing a ring, a thrift store ring with a fat, red stone in it. It sparkled under the soul-killing fluorescent lights. I fisted my hand and raised it, so that the bauble caught the light and tossed it in this little monster's face.

"I am a Satanist!" I proclaimed, there in my neighborhood McDonald's. "I Am a Satanic Witch. And I Curse You for Bothering Me. Your Dog Is Going to Die. It Is Done." I made a little flourish with my hand, the way I imagined a Satanic witch would cap off a dog-murdering hex.

I didn't know if this kid had a dog, *or did I?* The way his eyes grew large and filled with fear affirmed the chance I took was paying off. I raised my fisted hand, as if my ring was shooting an invisible beam of dog death at him.

"You better not!" he yelled, suddenly sounding like a kid, not a perpetrator. "That's horrible. You better not kill my dog!"

"It Is Done," I said mysteriously, and went back to my book. They stared at me, the small group of them, and shuffled out of the fast food joint, murmuring with alarm.

My first hex! I super-hope I didn't hurt that kid's doggy, as I love kids and love all animals. I always let spiders out onto my front lawn when I find them in the house, and my diet is a constant struggle between doctors telling me how nutrient-deficient I am and the heavy way consuming meat sits upon my heart. I really, really hope I didn't harm the dog. *But.* But if the kid's dog was, like, really old, and was quite naturally on death's

door, and happened to take his final breaths—coincidentally!—
that night, after he'd harassed a lone female for looking different
than he'd been taught to think a female should look, and forever
more he was always superstitious and kept away from weirdos
of all genders, sparing them a tendency toward harassment that
unchecked might have blossomed into violence—well, then, I
believe that sweet doggy would be *happy* to lend his inevitable
death to the cause of put-upon misfits everywhere.

Welcome to hexing.

As there are witches who aim to do only "good," and warn
against the evils of hexing, there are also witches who preach a
"If you can't hex, you can't heal," philosophy, the thought being
that avoiding our shadow side limits our power overall. One of
the things I so value about a witchy spiritual path is that we are
not held to standards of "goodness." No authority will ever tell
us we've transgressed, are bad, must repent and do penance.
We're allowed to observe our lives and be our own authorities,
making judgment calls as needed. And sometimes the verdict
is: that person needs to be *stopped*.

As for the arguments against hexing, they're actually pretty
relatable—there's too much bad energy in the world, and
witches shouldn't be conjuring more. Witches, being special,
spiritual people, are more obligated to take a higher road in the
face of whatever ill we'd like to lash out at. Finally, there is the
infamous Wiccan "Rule of Three": whatever vibes you put out
into the Universe, you'll get back threefold. Such notions are
hard to argue with, and, as a pro-hexing witch, I'm not going to.
If you want to live in love and light 24–7, have at it. For me, one

thing that drew me to witchcraft as an oppressed teen (other than the, um, aesthetic) was that, unlike the Christianity I was raised with, there wasn't pressure to "turn the other cheek." I didn't want to turn the other cheek! I wanted to smack my bullies flat on *their cheeks*! And witchcraft, it seemed, gave such expressions of consequences and revenge the green light.

A few caveats about hexing. I *do* think it's pretty good practice to keep your side of the street as clean as possible— meaning, try not to be a petty, vindictive witch. If someone doesn't want to be with you, the truth might ache your heart and your ego, but none of us are required to be with any of us. Imagine if someone *you* didn't like sent punishing rays your way because you simply weren't attracted to them? It would feel pretty unjust. For me, this notion of *justice* is what guides me in my hexing. If someone is within their rights and I happened to get butt-hurt because I didn't get what I thought I wanted, well, tough titties. I personally don't want to annoy the Goddexx asking for her help in fighting my punier battles. But, there are enough serious battles facing us that anyone who wants to give a hex a holler will find no shortage of deserving marks.

In my early twenties, a good friend who had gone to a party reported the next day that she'd been assaulted. A guy had followed her into the bathroom and shoved his hand down the back of her pants while trying to kiss her. She fought him off and left the apartment, but she was shook by the experience. At the time, I had put down my witchcraft practice and was devoting all my energy to direct action: protecting abortion clinics, marching with Queer Nation, lending my body to ACT UP die-ins. I also liked to come up with my own little protests for smaller targets: disrupting a mass at a church whose pastor tried to rally his congregation to besiege women's health clinics; causing chaos in a shop that had specifically stated they wouldn't hire gay people. I had a tight band of like-minded, angry friends— not unlike a coven, actually—and we set about finding a way to frighten this man with some consequences. We devised a complicated but effective ruse that allowed one of us to enter his home as a "journalist," leaving the door unlocked; the rest of us soon poured in, chanting and hollering, filling his apartment with our wild, angry energy. The action was half quasi-criminal vigilantism, spray-painting his name and his crime on the sidewalk outside his house, and it was half spiritual vengeance. One of us, a tall, long-haired woman named Lynn Alice Liberty, kicked the man's mattress as we paraded through his room, doing a quick little thing with her eyes, mouth, and hands. "I hexed his bed," she explained later. "He'll never be able to get it up there again." I gaped at her, delighted. I hadn't known she was a witch! We really *are* everywhere, I mused, excited at the thought of combining my new passion for direct action with my enduring devotion to this ancient spiritual practice.

And this is mostly the role hexing has in my practice: rather than curse the children who might gawk at my style, I'm more likely to direct such energies toward the larger sociopolitical ills we face. And from a glance at the media, I know I'm not alone. Scrolling through news, you'd think witches did nothing *but* hex Republicans! Which would be *fine*. Such hexes are, I think, a great way to do *something* with all that pent-up anger and stress and ennui and despair we so often get when we survey the landscape. It doesn't take the place of actual activism, of course—we still have to get out into the street and wave our signs and, Goddess help us, *chant*—but it feels good to do something energetic with all the cultural yuck. For instance, just yesterday, I finished working on this chapter for the day and got ready for a small march and rally happening in my neighborhood. Like many spots in the United States, my local school board is being targeted by fascists who are so upset about *rainbow flags* (is there nothing more benign?) being hung in school during Pride Month that they've taken to doxing teachers, making outrageous and grotesque accusations against queer allies, and bringing deeply grim "straight pride" flags and comically oversize MAGA hats to impromptu rallies. Some pro-queer parents had organized a little march to the school board's meeting, where the public comment session had been drawing crowds of bigots for months. I was happy to put my body out there to help raise the numbers. The last few times this had happened, the anti-queer contingent was bigger, louder, more organized. The bigots had recruited hateful people from spots all over Southern California, mostly men, and they carried expensive sound systems and had vans and trucks wrapped in hateful messages, just driving around my neighborhood, inspiring fear and discomfort in queers and allies around town. Of *course,* I'd be there. I was even prepared to (gag) *chant* if asked: "The people! United! Will never be defeated!" Or, "What do we want? Justice! When do we want it? Now!" If I was lucky, we'd just have a good, old-fashioned ACT UP "Shame! Shame! Shame!"

The rally was meeting up in a parking lot outside a Cost Plus World Market, then marching together the five or so blocks to the school board. The absurdity of a bunch of suburban Los Angeles queers and allies meeting up in a strip mall—close to the local Michaels, where many craft queens bought their glue guns—was not lost on me. Reviewing the text I got about the action, I noticed some reverends from a groovy, inclusive Christian church scheduled to speak at the top of our procession. I wondered how I might be able to bring my own spiritual practice into the mix. Of course—I should perform a little hex at my altar before marching out the door!

I had just the thing: a weird candleholder that legit looks like a penis, gifted to me by a friend as a joke (I presume?). It perfectly fit a black votive candle. Black, excellent for binding energy, for absorbing negativity, for conjuring power, for fighting. I took some Dark Moon tincture made by a witch I love, Dori Midnight, and anointed the candle with it. Anointing candles with oils and tinctures that correspond with your intentions is another way to oomph up the power of the ritual, bringing in some more magical actors to work toward your purpose. I chose this Dark Moon potion because the dark moon is secret, and powerful, and the moms organizing this march had deliberately kept the information off social media. Word of it traveled by text, from trusted ally to trusted ally. I thought of the many activists who had been showing up at recent rallies in hoods and face masks, dark sunglasses and wide hats, laboring to conceal their identities from the homophobes prone to doxing. I asked the Goddexx—Hekate, specifically, as she is a Witch Queen who is down to hex—to protect all her children and keep them safe, let them move in the shadows to do her work, if needed. I lit the candle and thanked other deities who had come through in recent tarot readings, whom I had made offerings to on my altar—would they lend their passion and hard work to this fight? What I was asking for, in general, was for the antis to fail. For them not to be successful. For today not to go in their favor, and for those on the side of queer and trans kids to be strong and powerful and triumphant. I spritzed myself with some of Dori Midnight's Boundaries in a Bottle, popped an obsidian in my tote for protection, and left the house.

An hour later I was in front of the school board, surrounded by queer people and those who love them, everyone holding rainbow pinwheels, opening rainbow parasols against the sun, tying pride flags around their necks like superhero capes. The antis were, for the first time in months, nowhere to be found. Some said it was because the march had been promoted Dark Moon style, whisper to whisper; others guessed they were, sadly, rallying in some other community that night. I didn't share that a tiny, burning candle and a plea to some cosmic icons *might* have helped, but I was deeply pleased. So pleased I didn't just chant with my fellows, I *sang*. Along with the gay preacher leading the song, I stood outside the school board and sang Bob Marley's "One Love" with a crowd of folks who, like me, had been needing a peaceful, feel-good win.

Other times, a hex might not give you what you want but what you need. I was once out of my mind "in love" with a charismatic Gemini. I put quotes around "in love" because, was I? Or, having been recently flung back into the dating world by my newly opened marriage, was I simply awash in chemicals, my dormant sex addiction surging? Either way, I was certainly out of my mind. My crush was being plagued by an old ex, a femme who kept showing up at the bar where he worked radiating bad vibes, saying curt things to him on group-text threads. You know, *twenty-something drama*. I was certainly too old to have an opinion about it all, but I was "in love," and these things were giving my frazzled Gemini amour *nightmares*—certainly, as a witch, I could do something about it? I decided I would bind the bad energies she was shading him with.

I learned about binding spells the way I've learned about so many spell practices, a mish-mash of occult books I've been reading and reviewing for decades. My first was *The Modern Witch's Spellbook;* my most recent is Judika Illes's mammoth *Encyclopedia of 5,000 Spells.* There is also, you may have heard, this thing called the internet, where bazillions of spells recipes and inspo live. I find that if you seek and study and practice for long enough, when the need for a quick-and-dirty spell hits you, you know just what ingredients to reach for.

The banishing spell was actually quite an enjoyable activity. We were in a long-distance affair, and I was frequently filled with an urgent yearning that I didn't know what to do with; crafting some witchery felt like a good action to take. I went about sourcing materials for a classic binding powder, scraping sulfur from match heads and adding it to a spice bottle filled with hot pepper and dirt from my yard. I added salt, added garlic. I crumbled a bay leaf. I shook it all together, the ghastly, nasty crumble taking shape inside the jar. On a piece of paper I wrote my Gemini's ex's name again and again, chanting, "I bind your energy from harming Charismatic Gemini." When the paper was full, I knocked some of the powder onto it and folded it up. Outside in my yard, in the dark, I buried it in the dirt.

Did the ex leave my Gemini alone? I don't know; we broke up shortly after. While our relationship had some incredibly high highs, it was at core pretty toxic. I like to imagine the Universe sussing me out, like, *Okay, you summoned me here to help this fuck boi you caught feelings for, but* you *seem like the one who needs some help right now, so let's just cut this cord.* I've had spells go sideways on me like this before, like the time I and a coworker-witch sprinkled some of our urine in the corners of a particularly awful boss's office. Within a month we were both, thankfully, gone from that job. I'm grateful to the Universe for giving me not what I want, but what I need. I like knowing that I'm free to ask for whatever I desire, knowing Spirit, their eye on a picture too large for me to grasp, will make the final call. Either way, a certain prayer is answered.

If you want to stay away from hexing because it just doesn't feel right to you, you should follow that. If hexing and cursing *do* feel right for you, have at it. Do try to keep your side of the psychic street clean; wasting the Universe's energy on petty grievances just seems misdirected, especially when there are more potent problems that could use your magic. If you are on the fence about whether to hex or not to hex, sample some of the following *hex lite* spells I've devised.

MARIE LAVEAU'S WITCH BOTTLE

Certainly you already know Marie Laveau, America's most famous witch. A voodoo priestess in New Orleans (a Catholic, as well), her life spanned nearly the entirety of the nineteenth century—and would have kept going, had her ploy to have her daughter pretend to *be* her after her death succeeded. Talk about a dynasty. A free woman of color from birth, Marie Laveau was a descendent of enslaved Africans and French colonizers, a mother to seven children, a hairdresser, and a professional conjurer, offering ceremony and services including midwifery, herbs, and gris-gris (charms or curses) to the mostly female clientele who visited her at her home on St. Ann Street in the French Quarter. The summer solstice rituals she began over a century ago on the Bayou St. John continue each year, and indeed the city still reverberates with her energy and legend, whether through touristy tchotchkes or the offerings left at her grave in St. Louis Cemetery No. 1.

One of the things I do like about voodoo is that it does allow for hexing and cursing and getting revenge; I can't help but admire practices that allow us to be our messy human selves. I say this even as I put in time every day meditating with the hopes of elevating my consciousness—or maybe, I say it *because* I spend so much time trying to level up my higher self, only to find myself beset by familiar, petty emotions. Sometimes, I find, the key is to indulge those feelings, to ask the Universe to assist you in sourcing some accountability when its absence is driving you wild. And so, I've crafted a Witch Bottle spell in honor of Marie Laveau, who I'm sure doled out as many curses as blessings during her time on Earth.

Now, this nasty spell is for when someone really, really, *really* needs some bad luck to head their way. I'll trust that you will use it only for those humans whose ill intentions badly need to be thwarted. It's such a gnarly spell, I expect only the angriest, most vengeful witches will attempt it, and I can only imagine they have their reasons! The first thing you need is a bottle. I like glass, don't you? However, if you want to give a malefic second life to a bottle made of single-use plastic, I'd say you'd be doing a good thing. Now, first, you must pee into the bottle. Don't *fill* it with pee—I'd say just, like, an eighth to a quarter. Before you pee, get yourself really worked up into a vengeful state. Sort of like the opposite of meditation. Fill yourself with righteous rage and anger, and then pee all that fury into your bottle. Next, add some spices: chili, paprika, pepper of all sorts, ginger. If you have a chunk of ginger or actual peppercorns, use those. Add a squirt of lemon juice to the bottle. Next, deliver it to the vicinity of your nemesis. If you want to be super slick, do all this in a miniature way, in the sort of teeny craft bottles you can get at Michaels, and then toss it into your target's bag or pocket or home or office—go for it, maniac! Otherwise, try burying it on their property, or as close to their property as you can get. Toss it in their bushes? Sure, just get it near them, and be however daring you can manage to be in the process. Then, go home and take a nice, soothing bath, and try to let go of all those hot, heavy emotions. You did what you could, now let it go. Release your energetic connection to this bozo, and watch it spiral down the drain with your dirty bathwater when you're done.

HEKATE'S HEX TABLET

Did you know that archeologists have found ancient hexing spells in Grecian ruins? Some are complex, like the earthenware jug found near the Athens Agora, stuffed with chicken bones and pierced with a nail; others, like the one found at the mouth of a well in downtown Athens, is just a simple slab of lead cursing the vagina of a newly married, and hotly envied, bride. If you are into ceramics and pottery and want to craft yourself a bespoke cursing jug to stuff with the remnants of last night's roast, well, I'm in awe of you. The rest of us will take the path of our petty friend downtown and fashion ourselves an angry slab.

Our curse tablet will be made of salt, which is way better than lead for the obvious reason no one gets poisoned, as well as the additional magic properties salt will super-charge your slab with. Grab a cup of flour, a half cup of table salt, and a half cup of water. Mix together until it's nice and smooth, then roll it out with a rolling pin. Using a sharp object—a pin or letter opener or X-Acto knife—carve your curse into the wet dough. Name names (but not your own!). Ask for what you would like to see happen. It can take up to seven days for salt dough to dry, so leave it someplace private where it won't be discovered or disturbed during this period. Once it's hardened, bring it to either a body of water, or to a cemetery—these are the two spots where ancient Greek and Roman witches liked to stash their curse tablets. In a cemetery, it will attract the spirits of the dead, who are psyched to lash out at the living who are wasting their precious human lives making this place miserable for the rest of us. Do speak aloud and ask whatever spirits might be hanging about if they mind doing you a favor and helping you curse a creep. Same goes for the water. There is an ancient belief that spirits move through water, so once again, if you drop your spell by a river or reservoir, see if anyone is around and open to doing your bidding. Don't forget to say thank you.

CELTIC CURSE BOWL

You might know that the entrances to many churches have little stone fonts filled with holy water for congregants to bless themselves with before they stroll into a pew. You probably won't be *terribly* surprised to learn that this is an appropriated Celtic pagan tradition, a riff on the rock bowls known as bullauns. Bullauns can be large boulders, or they can be stones that fit in your pocket, but what makes a bullaun a bullaun is that the rock has an indentation on its surface that forms a little cup or bowl able to hold a bit of water (and the larger bullauns may also hold additional stones in their curve). In ancient times, bullauns could be used to curse, but only if the curse was truly justified and pure. No cursing a rival's vagina here!

To find yourself a bullaun, go out to the shore, or to a rocky part of earth, and start looking. You might not find one, but if you do, won't you feel lucky? For those city witches who don't actually *know* where to find a bit of rocky nature (I feel you, sister) make yourself a faux bullaun with a bit of air-dry clay and some liquid epoxy resin (take care that you don't accidentally buy resin that requires a UV light cure, unless you're some sort of wild epoxy pro).

- Shape your ball of air-dry clay (found, again, at a craft store or internet supermarket) into a somewhat organic, rock-like shape.
- Next, make an indentation in it, a nice deep one. Like the salt dough, the air-dry clay may take up to a week to dry. Keep checking on it until it's no longer damp to the touch.
- When it's ready, take your liquid epoxy resin, a two-compound substance you'll have to mix together, and pour it over your bullaun. Make sure you don't fill up your indentation with the resin; it's okay if it pools in there a bit, but you want there to be room for your unholy water. It will take about a day for the resin to dry.

Now you've got your unnatural, DIY bullaun, perhaps made even *more* powerful by the work you put into making it. On that tip, regard the entire construction of your bullaun as a ritual;

light candles, burn things that smell mysterious, set intentions. While bullauns are great for (honest, righteous) curses, they are also handy for blessings, and the philosophy of the bullaun sees the magic work done with it as two sides of the same coin.

So, your bullaun is ready and you're set to send some bad vibes out to ruin someone's day. Traditionally, it is recommended to fast before working with a bullaun, and to leave offerings for the spirits. I think spirits always love sweet things, so honey and sugar can be great, and there are traditions that offer cigarettes and booze as well. If you have an idea of who it is you're asking for help—a specific deity or ancestor—tailor your offering accordingly. If it is more open, just leave something sweet, or pretty, like a lovely piece of fruit or a flower.

Fill your bullaun with water. Holding it in your hand or upon your altar (or on the ground, if you are outside), turn it three times counterclockwise and speak aloud who you are cursing and why, and what you would like to happen. Address whomever you are asking, if you are asking for specific magical assistance. If you'd like to use the bullaun for blessing, fast and present an offering, and turn the stone clockwise as you speak aloud the name of the person you are requesting blessings for, and why, and how. It is said that rainwater that collects in a bullaun's pocket is great for healing; just be sure, if you're working with an epoxy resin bullaun, that you do not ingest the water—but use it for sprinkling, candle dressing, or some other purpose.

Interlude:
What Are We
Even Doing?

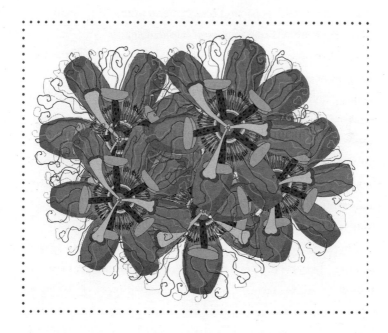

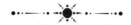

S omething happens when you are a mystical seeker. You do your meditations, only to feel your dumbass thoughts intrude, again and again, crashing into your attempts at emptiness. You stand before your altar, performing a ritual, only to not get the thing you were asking the Universe to deliver. You set intentions for the best part of your psyche to come to the fore, only to find yourself spying on your ex on the internet, or talking shit, or indulging whatever low-vibe compulsion you were begging the cosmos to eradicate. What are we meant to expect from this path? This phenomenon is important, because it often feels like *nothing* is happening.

Sometimes, when I probe a feeling of disappointment around my practices, I ask myself, *Well, what was I really hoping would happen?* and I realize, I want to feel high. And, while doing breathwork *does* sort of get me high sometimes, if you want to get high, you have to do drugs—and why am I looking to my magical practice for that experience? For some temporary relief from my dogged, earthbound humanity, duh. Well. Meditating and doing ritual is not going to get me high, and it's not going to turn me into a fairy. Bummer.

There is, nonetheless, a cumulative, if annoyingly glacial, positive effect on my personality, my ability to snag happiness or serenity, and, my favorite, a more frequent glimpse of the bigger picture. These flashes tend to come and go in a moment, but leave me bolstered with the notion that this world—the body

I'm in, the plain I exist upon, the way I perceive and analyze my life—is not all there is.

I have in my spirit a sort of auric spell bag, containing not rocks and herbs but memories, tiny insights I have gleaned from pursuing my interest in mystical things. I return to them when I feel lost or sort of blah, like nothing has any reason or sync, not my choices or circumstance, not my efforts or my nature. *What's the point?* is a common enough human query, and through working with magic, studying traditions, and allowing myself to believe in things unseen, I've come up with a grab bag of answers that don't exactly answer that unanswerable question, but do transform the attitude of the query from one of agitation to one of wonder. What *is* the point, indeed? Let's think about it!

Whenever I find myself taking things too seriously—feeling mournful that my "career" isn't in a different spot on the hierarchy of careers, glum that I haven't mastered capitalism, anxious with the thought of everyone's impending doom—I like to ask myself: What if everything was *exactly as it is meant to be?*

Easy enough for me to ponder, from where my safe, white body sits in a home, a plate of delicious food in front of me. This idea, that everything is meant to be, has certainly been abused by people with whom I have privilege in common. There are lots of new agey thinkers out there who have taken this thought and used it to blame victims, uphold systems of violence, validate atrocities. We live in a world that needs change desperately—racism needs to be eradicated, wealth needs to be redistributed, individuals need to be accountable for their often heinous actions. I don't believe that the poor, brown, queer, disabled people of this world are *meant* to suffer so much, any more than I believe that the wealthy, white, cisgender, able-bodied who hoard most of Earth's resources are meant to suffer so little. So how to square this faith that all is as it should be with the knowledge that things need to change, and we are meant to be agents of that change?

We've all heard that annoying F. Scott Fitzgerald quote about "first-rate intelligence" being the "ability to hold two opposed ideas in mind at the same time and still retain the ability to function." I don't want F. Scott or any dude mansplaining intelligence to me, and would much rather know what his wildling wife, Zelda, thought was a marker of a "first-rate" intelligence. But there is something to being able to sit with two very difficult, painfully opposed ideas: this reality is as it should be, and this reality needs to change. Let's hear from another writer, this one brown and queer, Rumi, and the phrase from his poem "A Great Wagon": "Out beyond ideas of wrongdoing and rightdoing, / there is a field. I'll meet you there." This piece gets blown around a lot on the internet, and I don't know that it's meant to suggest we all find someone diametrically opposed to our lives and go have a drink with them in a park. Part of my spiritual and political practice is to *not* try to talk sense to folks fighting against safe and legal abortion, or agree to disagree with folks whose response to Black people rising up in pain is "All lives matter." Nope. The verdict is out on whether this life I'm living is one of an infinity of lives, or simply my one precious life, but I am not going to waste the sand I've got left in the top of my hourglass to bang my head against *those* glass walls. What I take from it is that the Universe is vastly beyond the comprehension of the tools I was given to understand it. I don't understand how this place can be so gorgeous and so cruel; I don't understand how the most terrible things I can imagine have actually happened to actual people, and *still* this place has worth and meaning. Where I land with it is: I don't need to understand. It's quite beyond me. I only have to accept.

Acceptance can sound like forgiveness, something I find wholly overrated in spiritual communities. The idea that holding on to hurt and anger is toxic, the claim that healing cannot happen unless we drop our grudges, is as infuriating to me as the assertion that after death we all float up to a heaven in the sky to be judged by a bunch of white guys. Preposterous! Healing is individual and mysterious and almost certainly doesn't look or feel like what we might think it's meant to. Anger feels pretty crappy, it's true, but why do we think we're not supposed to feel crappy down here? In my own life, I have listened to people tell me that the holy, self-protective anger I felt at an abuser was *toxic*, by people who preferred to pretend the abuse never happened, and were made uncomfortable by the reminder of their own complicity. I've listened to people who betrayed me assert that until I stopped feeling bad about it I wouldn't feel better. There's a dumb logic in there—sure, I guess I *won't* feel better while I'm feeling bad, but I'm just going to hold a couple of opposing thoughts in my head and feel good about letting myself feel bad that I was treated poorly by someone I trusted.

I've wound up elevating the statement *I don't know* to a sacred utterance, a prayer, really, maybe even the core of my spiritual practice. It's a cosmic acceptance of the mystery in all of its confounding expressions, be it the zany design of a passionflower—those things are so bonkers, I could stare at them for days!—to the enduring riddle of why so many humans dedicate their lives to being against other humans.

Within *I don't know*, little glimmers about the nature of reality can make themselves known. Once, when I was in my twenties and reading a lot of mystical literature, always feeling on the cusp of knowing something, but never really getting it, I washed my hands at my sink. The stream of water was so clear it looked almost solid, like a *thing*, not liquid in motion. I pushed my hands into the stream, breaking it up into dozens of droplets. *That's us*, I thought, a moment of clarity hitting me. We are the mass of water, together, and we are the individual droplets. Around this same time—a mystically fruitful moment—I walked through downtown San Francisco, an area that was filled with people: businesspeople and unhoused people, spare-changing punks and skateboarders, robed monks and cops on bikes. And I thought, *We have bodies so that we can* experience *the particularity of all that is, instead* of being *it*. Like most mystical thoughts, it made a certain, revelatory sense in my body but it just sounds kind of stoner-y when you say it out loud. Still, it feels worth the attempt. I suddenly understood, just a smidge, the Buddhist concept of "no self." I called myself *Michelle*, and I had a lot of thoughts about myself—a seemingly unstoppable, endless flow of them, actually—and I looked a certain way and believed that physicality is also this thing, *Michelle*, but really, I am a shard of a universe smashed into a bazillion discrete pieces.

I am not *Michelle* at all. And my life may make a limited sense here, as a solitary thread, but it really makes sense when I come together with all that is unknowable, the giant everythingness of the Universe.

I can't unthink this thought, and it has brought me strange comfort. Sometimes I witness a person who just seems horrible. We all do, right? If we watch the news or listen to murder podcasts or even just coexist among humans, we confront the existence of people who are just awful. I think of them as a shard, a particular shard, of the Universe's many and mysterious energies. Maybe it would all feel so different were we to all be as one, all of our discrete energies overlapping and merging. Maybe in some other realm it is so, and we feel it, like a constant, freaky orgasm. But here I am only this, and my purpose in this life is to experience what it is to be this particular shard of the whole, this particular combination of energies. And to witness, from the outside, what the other energy combos can be, and think that the Universe is a great and terrible place, where everything that can exist, does.

Once, on an airplane—I have a lot of mystical thoughts on an airplane. Do you?—I looked around at all the humans and imagined us as fingers in a glove. Individual, yet not—a revelation that allowed me to see our seamless connection. Since then, I've conjured a bit of this cosmic, unconditional love when in public in a different way: I'll look at a stranger and imagine myself walking alongside them, my arm slung around their neck or waist, like a dear friend. It fills me with a friendly feeling, and challenges any aversion I might have felt toward the person, conscious or unconscious. Like a lot of white Americans, my first introduction to Buddhism was through the writings of the white, American Buddhist nun Pema Chödrön. *Drop your preferences* was one of her lessons; *drop the storyline.* Chödrön learned this concept from her own teacher, the fascinating and controversial Chögyam Trungpa, whose classic, *Cutting Through Spiritual Materialism,* is a warning about how spiritual practices, like everything else in life, can be weaponized by our stealthy egos if we aren't aware. "We can afford to surrender that raw and rugged neurotic quality of self, and step out of fascination, step out of preconceived ideas," he writes.

It's a powerful thing to practice, since most of the time we feel like we are nothing *but* our preferences and storylines, our preconceived ideas. But when I want to glimpse that part of me that is *not* Michelle, that aspect of mind that sees past this shard of me into the grander vision of *we* helps, dropping my preferences and storylines, especially when it comes to other humans.

Wait. You bought a book about witchcraft, something I'm more or less qualified to write about, and now you're getting all this Buddhism, something I am admittedly *not* qualified to speak on. But I've imagined this work as an investigation into what a/my solitary magical practice looks like, and in my case, it is very influenced by the magical gleanings I received courtesy of my forays into that practice. It greatly informs the sort of witch I am, the witchy thoughts I have and the rituals I do. Mostly it has given me tremendous faith in the Universe, that there is so much more than I can see, and that there is goodness in it, a goodness I can trust and work to grow within myself. Once, while flying in a plane—again!—we started to experience turbulence. As the plane began to shake and bounce, I felt the immediate sting of panic, and I began to respond as I always do, getting all clenched up, praying in my head a backbeat of sadness that I was obviously about to *die!* But then something occurred to me. It came from my immersion in Buddhism, from thinking about time, mindfulness, *the NOW.* If time was an illusion, and all there really ever is is *now*, and *right now* I'm fine, not dying, not dead, then couldn't I just stay calm and awake within the *Now*, regardless of the phenomena that it brought me? I took a deep, shaky breath. I opened my eyes. The plane kept rumbling. *Now* I was fine, alive. And *now*. And *now*. At some point that will change—what will the *Now* feel like then? Instead of afraid, I felt curious. For a moment, death didn't feel scary; instead, it felt truly like a sort of entrance, a massive set change, a total mystery but one I could remain conscious for, and face with eyes open.

All of this casts an interesting shadow in my magic practice. It has made meditation part of that practice. That part of me that knows it's wearing a *Michelle Tea* suit and playing a particular role in spacetime; that is who I try to locate when I make magic. If I'm wanting something so badly I want to cast a spell for it, I think about what would happen if I *dropped my preferences*, and see how that changes my intentions. I almost always still do the spell—doing spells activates a particular part of me that feels good, and helps me talk to Spirit—but maybe it becomes a bit more vague. Maybe I don't need *that producer to buy my idea for a TV show*; maybe I just need to ask that *my life continues to feel prosperous and adventurous.* I've learned to keep it open and trust that the Universe will fill in the details better than I ever could.

You have probably noticed what seem like contradictions in this chapter. I adamantly am not open to extending an olive branch to people who, for instance, protest libraries that host drag queen story hours. I also have practices that provoke feelings of unconditional love for humans. If my cosmic logline is *I don't know*, then my cosmic action is *both/and*. The Universe is literally everything, and that's a lot for my puny, little glorified monkey brain to comprehend. Thankfully, I don't have to figure any of it out to have a solid spiritual practice. I can pray, *Thank you, for all of it,* while I light my candles of devotion; I can pray, *I don't understand*, when I learn of something painful, and let myself feel grief. I can pray, *I don't understand*, when I hear of something wonderful, and let myself feel joy. In the tarot, The High Priestess sits, calm, between two columns, one black, one white, representing duality, the *both/and* of life on Earth. Much of the tarot, and of ancient esoteric writings, speaks about duality, much of it clumsy, reduced to things such as "male" or "female." Again, our glorified monkey brains are only equipped to fathom so much. While I'm here, this little shard of the Universe made flesh, I will seek as much as I am able to, until I pass back over into oneness, where just maybe all my questions won't be answered so much as *known.*

RITUAL FOR HEIGHTENED CONSCIOUSNESS

Ask the Universe for how many days or nights you should do this ritual by taking a deck of tarot or playing cards and shuffle, asking this question. The numerical value of the card is your answer.

Set your altar with a candle or candles—shades of purple and indigo are good, as are white or black, and silver or gold. There are so many crystals that are cool little helpers for expanding consciousness: all forms of quartz, amethyst, calcite, fluorite, and petrified wood are some that are easy to find and pretty affordable. If you're spendy, moldavite has a lot of this power. You can also work with copper, which amplifies the powers of whatever crystal it's near.

If you happen to be friends with a local birch or oak tree, grab a twig or leaf. If not, pull some marjoram from the spice rack. I like to make an offering of it on my altar and prepare of little cup of it as a tea, even though it tastes a little funny. Gardenia and lotus are also helpers, whether you have access to actual petals or maybe just some oil.

Burn frankincense. If you have a doggy familiar, bring them into the space with you. If you have an owl or raven feather, place it on your altar. If there is a deity you connect with who rules over higher thought, enlightenment, and/or death, make them an offering. Now, you're going to meditate.

I like to hold stones in my hand when I do this sort of meditation. I also set a timer from a meditation app, so I'm brought out of my trance with something nicer than a manic beeping. Set yourself up, get comfy, and just breathe. See if you can detect a sensation, a bit of energy at the crown of your head. We all have energy vortexes that line our auric bodies; Indian mystics began working with them over 3,000 years ago, naming them chakras. While the Hindu tradition holds the most knowledge about this incredible part of our selves, it is not my tradition, and has been pretty bastardized by white Westerners like myself who grasp on to just a piece of what is a vast, complicated, and entwined practice. I neither want to appropriate the Hindu understanding of these vortexes, nor do I want to ignore the fact that this enormous contribution to mysticism is the work of millions of Indian seekers. So. I say this, and I say that I can feel the whirling at the top of my skull when I bring my attention to it in meditation, and I do believe it is a place where I am able to receive divine energy. Rays from the Universe, Aquarian downloads from space, maybe just energetic waves that are all around us all the time, but we can feel it and become more conscious about calling it in through this vortex.

So, do it. Sit, meditate. You will be annoyed—your brain is a thought-producing machine and it will continue to do its job, pumping stupid little thoughts into your consciousness. Just wave them away and try not to make too big a deal about it. This process, done regularly, will give you some pretty great insight into the nature of your thoughts, which is, you should ignore most of them. Of course, you will likely get some more meaningful thoughts from meditating as well, so keep a journal handy for when you come out of it.

Meditating, just breathing. Sensing the energy at the top of your skull and breathing into it. Trusting that your intention to become more conscious about reality, whatever that might mean for you, does not have to be vocalized or encased in language to be known, that you are embodying this intention, that your actions are the intention. To be more aware of the flow of life around you, to be more cognizant of synchronicities, to be more open and available to the flow of life around you in all its glory and monstrosity, to be devoted to being alive and curious about all we can't fully see with our physical senses. Sit as long as you like. I usually aim for 15 minutes. And repeat as the tarot advised. Speaking of tarot, the heightened state you'll be in post-meditation is great for reading cards.

COOKIE + FRIENDS CHOSEN ANCESTOR MEDITATION

The point of this reading and meditation is to make contact with a chosen ancestor. We all know about the idea of our DNA ancestors around us, waiting to be called upon to guide us in this life. I like that idea, too, and do think that my grandfather and maybe grandmother have been with me. But, though I love my family of origin, as a queer person and general misfit I have always looked to nonfamily members—artists, legends, and icons from history who I've felt a kinship with—as inspiration and a way of locating myself in spacetime. If we can have chosen family in our lives, why not chosen ancestors? I often reflect on the bold and incredible lives of queers and feminists who came before me; it can really help when the problems of my own place and time feel so suffocating that my very spirit sags. Situating my own humble life on a continuum with these geniuses—recognizing that no matter how rough things feel, they had it harder, and it was their labors that make my own experience relatively smooth—this puts things in perspective. It also triggers gratitude, and a feeling of being beloved. Wouldn't these queer and feminist ancestors be so happy to see how I thrive? Also, OMG, I thrive! Thank you, ancestors.

As part of a workshop I once conducted, I, along with a Zoomfull of others, set about locating who I would like my chosen ancestor to be, and respectfully requesting that they walk with me in my life. Some participants didn't know who they wanted to ask, and so they hit the internet in search of people from history who shared some strands of their intersectional identities: queer poets, feminist anarchists, etc. I myself felt drawn, in my gut, to Cookie Mueller, the actress, writer, and adventurer who starred in John Waters's early films and whose autofiction and advice for drug users is published in the collection *Walking Through Clear Water in a Pool Painted Black*. I chose Cookie because she was queer, having had important relationships with both dykes and straight men. She was a mom. She spent significant time in Provincetown, a spot I also feel a connection to. She was a Pisces, and my birthday falls on the day the sun moves from Aquarius to that water sign. She was wild, truly wild, during a time when it was much harder, more punishing, to be a reckless, adventuring female. She did drugs and hitchhiked and fell in love and got her heart broken, gave birth and made iconic art and wrote about it all. And she was witchy, of course, always with a crystal in her purse and a compassion so mystical that she once cried at the New England Aquarium after hearing some Massholes talk shit about an octopus. An IV drug user, she died of HIV in the 1980s, her death documented by her friend the photographer Nan Goldin. Cookie was an iconic art maker even in death.

The first thing I did was a meditation, asking the spirit of Cookie Mueller to connect with me. You can do the same with your chosen ancestor. I did this meditation seated, at my desk, because I wanted to quickly write down all of the hits I got, messages, bits of communication. You have to trust yourself, that the messages you are getting are real. I thought this would be harder for me than it actually was; when I steadied myself and focused, I felt Cookie Mueller come in strongly. It immediately brought tears to my eyes. I felt a big sadness from her, which was unexpected; though she of course felt sorrow, I regard her as a joyful creature, but she wanted her sadness to also be known. She was sad, I felt, at being regarded as a "bad mother." She made a lot of parenting choices that I, and many parents, wouldn't make—choices I *do* tend to judge, if I'm being honest, but I never judged them in Cookie. She got the sort of pass I often give to artists and legends I admire—they were living on another level. Their art, and their eternal inspiration, excuses it. In my meditation, I felt her sadness at being judged, and the power of her love for her child. I held that love and honored it; it is the same love I have for my son. It felt familiar; even how it was laced with sadness was familiar. I felt Cookie's energy near me and breathed it in for a while, breaking out to take notes, but never losing the connection.

Then I did, and you will do, a tarot reading. Shuffle the cards and ask your intended if they will do this thing with you, be one of your ancestors, a spirit who is available to come to your psychic and emotional aid, to look out for you in this plain from the beyond. Then, lay out the cards:

Card 1: Why do you want to work with this spirit?
Card 2: Spirit's initial thoughts about this request
Card 3: What you should know about this spirit
Card 4: What this spirit should know about you
Card 5: How this spirit would be able to help you
Card 6: How you would be able to help this spirit
Card 7: Your answer

I was surprised at how sort of ornery Cookie's answers were. Again, everyone has moods, but I hold her as a bit of a gentle soul. I appreciated the fullness of her spirit coming through. I got a lot of "why me?" energy from the reading, not in a humble way but more of a "Why are you bothering *me* with this?" energy. She was not initially sure she wanted to do it; she was curious but also didn't want to get bogged down by me. I don't remember all the specific cards, but one was the Lust card in the

Thoth tarot. It's a card that really aligns with the way I regard her energy: a ferocious lust for life. Cookie loved being human. Though there are no doubt many people who call on her ancestral skills as actual family, as well as more who, like me, seek her as our chosen one, she would be up for it if I can bring more of that passionate, human lust for life her way, that fiery energy her moon in Aries fed upon. It's a tall order, my life these days being more geared to third-grade car pools than cross-country hitchhiking, but the challenge to make my life Cookie-worthy was her first gift to me.

I keep Cookie in all of my meditations and do offerings for her at my altar. I call upon her especially as a mother, because she was a powerful one. A good one. Your relationship with your own chosen ancestor will find its own expression; just be conscious of them in your magical workings and throughout your day.

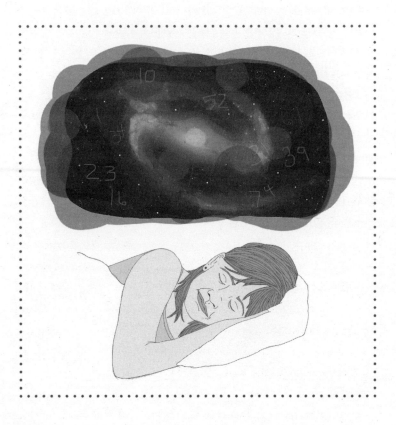

Dreaming Is Free

In her bedside table, my grandmother kept a very important book. Having lost its cover long ago, it appeared as
a slightly exploded-looking collection of ratty pages, the
corners flipped and slightly grimy. It was a book that had been
through a lot. Open it up and you'd see that the mayhem wasn't
confined to the tattered outside; the pages were heavily noted
in blue pen. This was my grandmother's *Lucky Numbers Dream
Book*, a compendium of every type of person, place, or thing you
might encounter in a dreamscape, and a corresponding number
for you to play in the lotto.

It might seem like a cheapening of dreamtime's mysteries
to put them to work for us in such a way, but my grandmother
grew up in a broke, abusive household, her sweet mom and
passel of sisters all at the mercy of the drunken patriarch. She

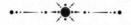

escaped that place and landed in a nurturing relationship with my grandfather—a happy-go-lucky Sagittarius who was disinclined to fighting, let alone abuse—but life was never financially easy. My grandfather dropped out of high school to serve in World War II, and from then on worked as a machinist. My grandmother ran a cash register at the department store downtown. This was what was available, and there wasn't much more. If you had dreams, literal or figurative, of pocketing a little extra cash, it would have to come from the lotto. Which, in my grandmother's time, was illegal.

This is how it worked: My grandmother, a dreamy Aquarius, awoke in the morning and worked to remember her dreams. They tended to be vivid, so it wasn't normally much of a chore; more often than not, the problem was a plethora of dream images to work with, too many images and their corresponding numbers. She was on the *beach* (319) and saw a *dolphin* (750) caught up in a *wave* (745). Oh, 745 was also her daughter's house number, so make sure to play *that* one, maybe place an extra dollar on it. My grandmother would scribble all this intel down in a notebook—a dream journal with ambition, basically—and pop it in her purse. At some point during the day, Johnny the Bookie would swing by her register at the department store. My grandmother would write down her numbers and hand the man a roll of dollars; the women who worked the register alongside her did the same. If she was lucky—and her dreams and her guide guaranteed her she would be, at least occasionally—Johnny would come by the next day with my grandmother's payout.

My grandmother experienced these dreams as a mystical

thing, a bit of magic. She's had the experience of having lightly prophetic dreams; watching the nightly news, a particular story would trigger a cascade of memory, and she'd gasp— she'd dreamed about this, last night! A witchy woman without a safe route to explore and own this aspect of herself, she leaned into dreams—something so common, so universal and daily, yet deeply mysterious, connected to a reality somehow beyond our conscious selves. When she hit the number because of a dream she had, it felt like the ultimate proof that there was more to life, that some benevolent energy was looking out for her, speaking to her psyche through images and symbols.

Lucky numbers dream books like my grandmother's originated in the northeast United States in the 1800s; although white and Black folks alike played the numbers, anti-gambling efforts of the era portrayed the game and its players via negative stereotypes of African Americans. The same publishers who put out books of racist humor soon were printing dream books attributed to "Aunt Sally," a chubby-cheeked, kerchiefed mammy figure, as well as other non-white races prone to exotic stereotypes, such as Mehemet Ali and Gypsy Witch; even Mother Shipton, a famous Anglo witch from England, was given "Oriental" knowledge. But, by the 1920s, Harlem-based psychics and entrepreneurs were publishing their own dream manuals and selling them locally, to the same clients who swung by for a fortune-telling or a candle spell. The reality was, white-run banks would not loan money to Black people, and playing the numbers was a legitimate way to maybe score the cash needed to survive and maybe thrive. The leading Black publisher of lucky dream books was Caribbean immigrant and Harlem resident Herbert Gladstone Parris. His books are still published today under his pseudonym Professor Uriah Konje; this was the book my grandmother worked with. My heart leapt when I found it on the internet, still in print. I ordered a copy, and for a week I lived as my nana did, jotting down my dreams upon waking, then seeking their numbers in the book—supplementing, when necessary, from the free, online versions now available.

I still remember the dreams I had the week after buying the book, since my experiment with witchy dream gambling relied on me paying so much attention to them. After falling asleep while watching Alejandro Jodorowsky's surreal *The Holy Mountain*, I dreamt of poop; another night I was stranded in rural Mexico, at a defunct train station. Every afternoon I walked to the Armenian grocer across the street and placed my hopeful numbers; "Good luck," the friendly lady who worked the register said as she pressed the printout into my palm, a benediction. I'm not as lucky as my grandmother, who "hit" often enough to have faith in the game. I won no money during my week of dream gambling, but appreciated the deeper connection to the ineffable—inspired by my witchy ancestor to mine my dreams for good fortune in my waking life, taking a chance on randomness and chaos.

Ancient Egyptians believed that dreams took place in the realm between life and death, and that dreams contained messages from the land of gods and spirits. The oldest recorded nightmare in human history comes from Egypt, circa 2100 BCE:

a man was haunted by a recurring dream of his father's dead servant creepily staring at him. The guy wrote a letter to his dad, also dead, for help. The ancient Greeks and Romans, influenced by Egyptian culture, continued the tradition of valuing dreams as complex sources of knowledge. Learning that these long-ago and faraway people also had dreams of *their* teeth falling out leaves me feeling connected to a collective unconsciousness that seems to transcend spacetime. Rather than write off such a classic dream as your basic anxiety dream, the ancients turned to a metaphor of the mouth as your environment, with your top row of teeth representing the people closest to you, and the bottom standing in for acquaintances and various NPCs. Your basic tooth-loss dream becomes something deeper to work out in a framework such as this.

We all know that dreams are tunnels to our subconscious, where we keep all the things we know but don't want to know that we know. Memories suffused with longing or distress, childhood fears; the source of all desire perhaps lives here. My sex dreams tend toward the comically absurd or embarrassingly desperate. One memorable night I experienced an actual orgasm from a dream in which I *hugged Ronald McDonald* in a dark garden full of broken Grecian statuary. I could write a book unpacking the imagery: Clowns! Tenderness! Spooky environment! For many years I dreamed I was in the same building as my deepest tweenage obsession, Billy Idol, and if I could only find him, I could have sex with him. I had these dreams regularly from age 13 till around age 48, when I finally met up with him on his astral tour bus and did the dirty. Was it worth the wait? Sort of! That the dream preceded the shift of my marriage status from monogamous to polyamorous, an era during which I slept with bunches of cisgendered men for the first time in my life, was not lost on me. It was a predictive dream, but I was more fascinated with how it was evidence of processes happening at such a deeply subconscious level, I was barely aware of them. The puzzle of how to work with attractions to cis men as a queer, feminist woman had apparently been occupying my psyche for decades, and Billy Idol was the pretty face of that dilemma.

Now, I don't only *believe* that my dreams contain hints about the future, I know it to be true. In my twenties I went on a doomed road trip. I didn't know it was doomed, but my companions were destined to fall out with one another, and I'd be forced to choose sides. Taylor, who owned the vehicle, was in unrequited love with Max, and Max's lack of interest provoked in my lovelorn friend a fierce bitchiness. By the time we hit New Orleans, the vibe was unbearable; Max opted to Greyhound back to California, and I felt compelled to travel back with him. The morning Taylor dumped us at the Greyhound station in the business district, I didn't know I was in for a low-key supernatural experience.

The very first night of our trip, the three of us had spent the night at Taylor's grandparents' house in the Midwest. It was the scariest night of my *life*, as I was stricken by sleep paralysis till the sun came up, a prolonged experience that inspired a lot of fear and confusion. At times it had felt like my soul was trying

DREAMING IS FREE

to leave my body, but not in a fun, let's-astral-project-and-fly-around-the-Eiffel Tower way. More in a *something is trying to steal my spirit* kind of way. This exhausting night of little sleep ended when I awoke from a rather mundane dream that had filled me with terror. The dream was a simple vision: the head of a man in a type of uniform not unlike a police uniform, with that shape of hat upon his head. He faced away from me, and then turned toward me, looked me in the eye, and began to speak. The dream had no audio; his mouth moved but I heard nothing. His expression was calm, friendly, maybe a little bored. There was nothing scary about what I was seeing, yet my body was gripped with an immediate panic, the sense that I was *not* supposed to see what I was seeing. A horrible wrongness, a transgression. Aware now that I was dreaming, I succeeded in shaking myself out of the vision, the night's paralysis gone now that the morning sun had risen. I told my travel comrades about my strange and creepy night over coffee, and put it out of my mind as we plotted our course through the South.

That truly fateful morning, as I waited in line to board my Greyhound bus, I watched my dream come true. The driver taking tickets, head cocked to speak to a coworker, finally turned to address me, and my sleeping vision solidified: that pleasant, calm face; his uniform cap on his head; his lazy drawl: "Your ticket, ma'am?" I was shook, stared at him a beat too long, pulled myself out of it before he asked if I was okay, and boarded my bus with goosebumps roiling my body. A part of me *knew* the road trip would take this unexpected turn—not just a vague, intuitive, hunch way of knowing, but a crystal-clear, *literal* way of knowing, as if the entirety of our lives is projecting on a screen somewhere, ultimately known and knowable, if only we were able to enter the theater.

I've told this story a lot, and have thought about it even more. Like the time I saw a ghost—for real—it helps me trust my sense that there is more to our reality than the mundane if beautiful world we inhabit on the daily. Whenever I think about it, I'm struck by that powerful sense that I was *not* supposed to see it. I believed I was hitting on a cosmic truth as real as the prophetic nature of the dream itself. But why? Is it that we're not, ultimately, equipped—physically, mentally, emotionally—to comprehend the nature of our existence, which this dream provided the tiniest hint of? Would it cause us to stray too far from the path of consensus reality, making life impossible, perhaps tragic for us and those who love us? Would it spoil the plot, thereby spoiling our ability to be surprised, for our soul to learn certain lessons? Are we trapped in a simulation, the fear I experienced part of my programming to not look too closely at the glitches? I could sort of believe any of it. What I do know is what my grandmother seemed to know, and what the ancients surely did—that our dreams may indeed be a surreal rehashing of events and anxieties, but they're all swirled together with something more as well, coming from a part of us that knows more than we think we do, where our connection to the mysteries of the Universe are strongest, wisest—prone, if we're lucky, to spitting out, every now and then, an uncanny gem for us to work like a mystical puzzle that reaffirms our belief in spiritual possibility.

A DREAM FOR ROSALEEN NORTON

Oceanic witch Rosaleen Norton seems to have been born a witch, back in 1917 in New Zealand, in the midst of a wild and thunderous storm; her apparent magical powers weren't something she worked to hone as an adult, but something that seemed to have defined her childhood. Rosaleen spooked her Christian parents with her early psychic gifts: dreams that revealed to her demons and otherworldly creatures, beings she eventually taught herself to visit with in waking life through meditation. She moved with her family to Sydney, and by her early teens she had been kicked out of school for sharing her visionary artworks with her classmates. By seventeen, Rosaleen was married and had been studying art formally for about three years, supporting herself by writing, drawing, and posing as an artist's model.

Rosaleen's teenage husband never came back from World War II; her mother passed away not long after. Both tragedies pushed the mystic deeper into her destiny as the Witch of Kings Cross, the red-light district she moved to in the wake of these losses. Continuing to make art, often in defiance of the prevailing censorship rules, Rosaleen also continued her occult studies, educating herself on the Kabbalah and Eastern forms of mysticism before discovering the magickal systems created by Aleister Crowley, in particular sex magic. Continuing to meditate and put herself into a trance state to channel visions, Rosaleen was visited

CC•••— •• 181 ••— ••))

by pagan heavy hitters such as the Greek goat-god Pan, precursor to the Christian devil, as well as the dark Hebrew goddess Lilith and the queen of the witches, Greco-Roman Hekate.

Understanding that altered states of consciousness were gateways to the realm of archetypes and inspiration, Rosaleen began to augment her journeys with LSD. By this time she had gained a bit of infamy, her penciled eyebrows in a perennial arch, her tiny bangs and classic witchy couture causing a stir in 1950s Sydney, as did her magic sex parties, provocative embrace of so-called debased practices, reclaiming of the insult "witch," and her paintings, which elaborated on her beliefs and practices with the additional glamour of demons and assorted Satanic imagery.

Rosaleen's first solo art show was subject to a police raid, the work destroyed for breaking obscenity laws, a charge that was eventually dropped, though there was no getting those paintings back. As strong and righteous a witch as she was, Rosaleen's artistic career suffered under the strain of chronic attacks, both from the law and in the media. Her art book, *The Art of Rosaleen Norton*, was banned in both Australia and the United States, and the legal attacks extended to her intimates, with her British lover and magickal partner Sir Eugene Goossens, an acclaimed composer, seeing his own career shot in the foot after he was busted over a thousand sex photos in Australia. A Libra—look how her life was marked by art and parties and love affairs!—she died at 62 from colon cancer, and left behind a legacy of art and magick that the world continues to catch up with.

This dream ritual is built in her honor. Create a small altar by your bed; whatever you place there, make sure there is a pen and paper, as well as any images of particular deities or entities you wish to commune with. Say a prayer to your desired archetype before you sleep, and ask them to come to you in the dreamspace. Alternately, you can launch an open call into the ether, asking whatever goddexxes who stay by you to reveal themselves in your sleep.

When you awaken in the morning, try not to open your eyes or spring out of bed. Stay as still as you can, grab your pen and paper, and write down your dreams with as little disturbance to your physical body as possible. Your body is holding onto the dream images in some fashion; shake your body and you might shake away those visions. If you've stopped remembering, gently roll over into another comfortable sleeping position and lie for a moment, seeing if that shakes loose any dream memories. When you feel you've remembered all you can, sit up and review your notes, rewriting them neatly while it's all still fresh. Do this every day for a period of time—a week, a month, the rest of your life—and investigate who comes to you. You may not know who they are immediately, so take note of any detail you recall. In my own practice, I've noticed my lazy, half-asleep brain tries to dissuade me from capturing details, telling me it's not important—but it almost always is! A particular color or object associated with a dream entity might provide clues to your dream deity's identity. If you want to go full Rosaleen with this ritual, don't only take written notes, sketch or paint what you see in your dreams. Drawing from this different side of your psyche may bring forth more recollections and sharper detail.

When you have started to build an image of a dream-visitor,

whether you know what deity it is or only have a shadowy idea, spend some time each day meditating on this entity, calling them toward you, asking for further information. Take notes of whatever came to you after each sitting. Rosaleen Norton's primary god was the bacchanalian god Pan, and she built her relationship with him through dreams, meditation, trance, and art. May this practice be as fruitful for you.

*If you're not interested in communing with otherworldly entities, but *do* want to get deeper into your dreaming mind for better self-knowledge and stronger intuition, simply adopt the above dream journaling technique, keeping paper and pen by your bed each night and recording your dreams each morning, with minimal physical movement.

DREAM INCUBATION

This nifty tool is similar to Rosaleen's catch-a-goddess dream work, but rather than pray to an entity before sleep, you assign your mind a task. For instance, you are working on a novel, and you find yourself stuck and blocked at a particular spot. Tell your brain you would like to solve this problem as you sleep, and fall into slumber thinking about it. Record your dreams in the morning in the recommended way. This can solve not only creative problems, but personal problems, relationship conflicts, even point your life in a new direction if you've lost your way.

House Work

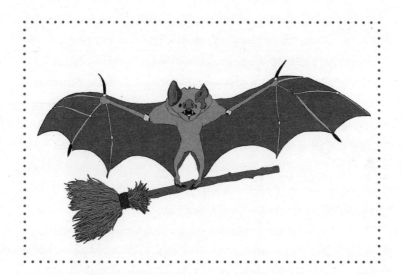

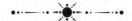

efore I moved into a sky-colored Victorian on a San Francisco side street, I'd shacked up with a girlfriend in New England, been run out of an obsessively communal Mission District walk-up, and had spent a couple of years living above an elderly alcoholic and below a trio of party kids who liked to roller-skate up and down their hallway, creating quite a racket. These homes all had their own energies, their own combo of roommates adding to the vibrational effluvia, but none of them were home for too long. Then there was The Blue House. It was there that I eventually had my name on a lease, triggering a deeply adult revelation: I'd been on my own, taking care of myself, paying rent on time for *years*. Sure, sometimes utilities were late, like when a dear friend on a bender stole our phone bill cash right off the table to buy drugs. And yeah, there was that time when the assemblage of roommates *were* a little short and had to throw a rent party, but we were always looking for a reason to throw a party, so you could hardly call that a problem. I remember my roommate Lucy, a loud, Leo Brit, drawing one of those fund-raising thermometers on the wall in the hallway, filling it in with red Sharpie as the party filled up. I remember bringing the wad of crinkly cash to the credit union and writing a check to Cort, our long-suffering downstairs neighbor *and* landlord, too kind to throw a bunch of feral twenty-somethings on the street no matter how many late-night after-parties had him banging on his ceiling with a broomstick.

I was surviving in The Blue House, but was I *thriving?* It's hard to say—my standards of living were so admittedly low (I preferred to think of them as *punk*), and I was so frequently so inebriated, I'm probably not the most reliable narrator of my own times. I loved the wildness the house seemed to radiate, calling toward it all the most random tenants. When I first arrived, I shared the space with a Thelemic witch and a belly dancer; when they moved out, I swiftly filled it up with a rotating cast of low-down queers: a vegan speed-freak math genius who alternated between debauchery and health kicks; a young lit student with a pet mouse; a sweet-smelling femme who cleaned up after everyone; a former crush whose back kept giving out; another former crush who suffered from depression and kept bringing home rescue dogs; a third former crush who had to cut off our friendship once she quit drinking; a stoner trance musician (plus her frequently homeless friend who was often snoozing on the couch); the newly sober psychic medium; multiple DJs, including the drug-addled one who'd hallucinated tiny police officers hiding under the living room chair; and the one who drank beer in the shower and moved her teenage runaway girlfriend in without asking. All of this energy would be enough, more than enough, but add to it the various lovers, girlfriends, and one-night-stands and the spikes of energy they brought in; the touring musicians I'd often find crashed out in my bed; and the after-party guests, with their energy-altering chemicals. I should not have been surprised when a psychic friend pronounced the place full of bad vibes.

Not vibes—*bats*, actually. The psychic friend who spied them was Meryl, whose band, Death Card 13, I played drums in. Meryl had years of sobriety under her studded belt. She was a butch rocker, Native American, and spoke with a Jeff Spicoli stoner-surfer drawl that belied her quiet wisdom. As I ransacked my fridge for something other than moonshine (for real) or Sunny D for us to drink (the Sunny D was possibly spiked), Meryl leaned against a wall, pensively staring at my ceiling, seeing something only she could see. Meryl had mystic abilities. "You got some bad-energy bats up there in the corners," she informed me, gesturing. I looked, but only saw the regular, billowing cobwebs. "Bats?" I clarified. Meryl nodded. "Yeah, they're up there, they're no good. They're probably throughout the house," she said, cocking her head as if calling forth the vibes elsewhere in the shotgun apartment. "You should clean," she suggested.

Ya think? Like everyone who ever lived in The Blue House (with the exception of the perfumed femme), I didn't care so much about cleaning. Entropy seemed to be set to fast-forward in that place, where so many people came and even more visited (once I arrived home after a bar closed to find a party in full swing, *but no actual tenants at home*); messes accumulated faster, and as we were all mostly always hungover, conjuring the energy to straighten up was arduous. It was easier to simply let your standards drop . . . and drop . . . and drop. When the rusted-out part of the shower floor grew too fearsome, I simply wore sandals in the shower to not cut my feet; when the drain became clogged, I brought in a milk crate to raise me above the waters. When the scent of dirty, musty clothes in my closet became too noticeable, I flung the clothes out my second-story window, ran down to the street to gather them, and lugged them to the laundromat. Sure, the trash at the top of the stairs grew large enough to be mistaken for a grisly art installation. Yeah, a roommate got a staph infection in her nose after wrestling with her boyfriend on our filthy kitchen floor (and yes, she passed it to me after we shared a rolled-up bill over a line of drugs). Somehow the claw-footed tub became filled with both dirty cat litter *and* dirty dishes (one or the other I could have maybe understood); somehow, the fungus we found growing on a dirty towel under the bathroom sink could not be identified by the academic mycologist we shared it with. Meryl was right—we *should* clean. But at that point, the grime in The Blue House was practically sentient, gaining consciousness as I did my best, day by day, to obliterate my own.

You should clean. These three words were powerful, but I wasn't spiritually ready to clean anything when I heard them. I found it easier to adapt to the consequences of the way I lived than to access the bird's-eye view needed to see what was really going on: that I was an alcoholic. That I let fantasies about sex and love get me wrapped up with people I was better off without. That the way I romanticized the bad behavior of infamous male writers was justifying self-destruction that came more from my alcoholic genetics than from the Beats. That I had an *inner child* (barf!) who needed some actual love and care. Like, nourishment, a bedroom that was *not* littered with moldy coffee cups, a shower that didn't risk a visit to the ER.

A different person in a different place might have received

Meryl's suggestion as a wake-up call and gotten serious about tearing the cobwebs from the corner, sweeping the cigarette butts off the floor, washing the grime off the windows, and maybe even talking to the kindly landlord about the basic unacceptability of a rusting, rotting shower. A different person would have perhaps taken a long, hard look at how she'd let her standards, her *self*, fall, and accept the challenge of climbing out of her toxic slump. But I had more years of drinking and using ahead of me, more bottoms to collapse into before understanding that beneath every bottom is yet another, more troubled bottom.

I believe that, much as our physical bodies have immune systems to help keep us healthy and strong, so do our psyches, or auras, or whatever you want to call the ethereal energy field that surrounds us (I once experienced my own as a bubble). Frequently, the same things that wear down your immune system—malnutrition, ingesting dirty drugs, saturating your body with alcohol, repeat exposure to pathogens—also weaken your psychic immune system. The longer I lived at The Blue House—I was there for seven years—the more the mess piled up, the more the negative energy accumulated, the more spiritually sick I became. With the healthy constitution of an able-bodied twenty-something, my body could miraculously bounce back, binge after binge. But, energetically, I became haunted.

There were multiple nights when I felt I was in a battle with a nefarious entity when I ought to have been sleeping. Mornings after these struggles were confused and confusing—did that all really happen? Was it a dream? Was it a dream, but *real*? As my alcoholism progressed, late-night fights with dates became normal, filling my little bedroom—whose walls I'd strewn with chunky ceiling glitter, cheerful whimsy I'd hoped would drive the bad-energy bats away—with even denser vibes. My inherent affinity for all things occult did not vanish during this time; it flourished, meaning I was playing around with spells and concepts when I was very much not grounded, losing touch with my own essence a bit more each day.

A witchy friend scolded me during this time, after hearing about my recurring (and terrifying) instances of sleep paralysis, the sense that something evil was in my bed with me. "You don't protect yourself," she said bluntly. She told me to spend time surrounding myself in white light and asking for protection, something I didn't do. Was *white light* possibly racist? I didn't want to take the chance. Plus, I was super into embracing the world as the unsafe place it was; rather than delude myself with the illusion of protection, I chose to hope that any demonic forces or gnarly ghosts hanging out around me chose to see me as a kindred spirit.

Eventually, my house began to scare me. I couldn't put my finger on it, but I could feel it, strongly: an energy that made me unwilling to walk down my long, shotgun-style hallway after dark alone. That hall connected my bedroom to the communal spaces and bathrooms: one water closet, one room with the rusting shower and the fungal towel, and an outrageous third bathroom with the litterbox/dirty dishes bathtub and a second toilet. It was that room—wide, painted red—that felt like the energetic nexus of the house's haunting, where maybe the

queen bad-energy bat haunted the corners with her volumi-
nous wings. If I had to go to the living room or kitchen after
dark, I'd make my boyfriend come with me; after all, he did
the same. The hallway and the big, red bathroom freaked him
out, too. If there was no escort available, I'd run.

It took years after this creepy experience to understand
that the house was trying to get rid of me. It wanted me gone.
When the thought occurred to me, it landed with a physical
force that gave me chills. It was time to go. Leaving was a terrifying thought—my rent was only $200, same as when I'd
moved in seven years hence. I'd never be able to find such a
cheap room again; my poverty mentality had me believing I
couldn't support myself anywhere *but* The Blue House. Probably
I accepted, even cultivated, the rock-bottomness of the environment because I believed I couldn't make a nicer place, with
higher rent, work. While I'd once patted myself on the back for
always paying rent on time, the reality was I didn't know how
to live as a functional, healthy adult. The bad-energy, dysfunctional vibes of The Blue House was all I could manage.

We all know that spaces hold energy. You may not have been
a guest at a Blue House party (or maybe you were—hi!), but
you've probably been in hotel rooms or other spaces that made
your skin crawl. Likewise, you've also surely been in environ-
ments that warmed you, that felt calm and nurturing and good
to be in. Even folks skeptical about other unexplained phenomena cosign the palpable spirit some places emit—scientists,
for example, have studied this curiosity, and have found a
possible explanation in *chemosignals*, the chemicals present in

sweat that may be detectible on a subliminal level. Emotions such as joy or fear can be transmitted in our sweat, and linger in a space after we've taken our sweaty bodies elsewhere. When you think about the number of highs and lows, so many of them chemically assisted, being experienced in The Blue House, by such a variety of people, and then, the house was *never cleaned*— why, yes, it might have just been all of us humans creeping one another out with pheromones we'd been littering the joint with like ashes off the end of a cigarette.

I don't know that I ever chose to leave The Blue House as much as The Blue House wanted me gone. An energy, a creepy vibe, seemed to be increasingly present in my home. I couldn't help but feel that the house had a spirit, and the spirit was over my bullshit. At the time I had fallen head over heels for a sullen, unemployed *teenager* (18, okay, but still, OMG; I might have been *living* like a teenager, but I was actually 27). This individual still lived at home, as so many teenagers do, and so he all but moved into my home. My roommates did not judge our age difference—queers age differently than the general population, as our dating habits sometimes prove—but they did *not* love finding this freeloading slam poet (yes) spending his afternoons watching *Unsolved Mysteries* on our pirated cable. The vibes grew tense. I tried to keep us confined to my bedroom, which is why I wasn't consulted on the decision to paint the living room a dingy sage green I found utterly depressing. I think that my roommates had, in their own way, each been reckoning with the bad-energy bats flapping around the house, and were trying to do *something* to banish them. I think the house itself felt the same. I think that it's entirely possible that *I* was the creatures' primary energy source. When an old friend called trying to convince me to move to Los Angeles, offering me a studio apartment in a building being managed by a mutual friend, I packed up my young lover and headed south. In Los Angeles, I felt inspired by the chance to start over in a new, clean apartment; the ways my drinking sabotaged my best efforts at a fresh start would slowly—sloooowly—become apparent, providing the impetus to eventually get sober.

Now, don't get me wrong—I'm still a slob. The desk I currently type at is strewn with tarot cards and scrap paper scrawled with notes, pens, and crystals and hand cream and stickers and knickknacks. A stack of unpaid bills stares me down from my windowsill (I'll be tending to them right after I finish this chapter). My eight-year-old son has to nag me to clean the cat box; a Libra, he will brush his teeth in the hallway if the smell gets too pungent. I'm not proud of any of this, and I always strive to Do Better, but my son has no idea how far I've come. The mess in my living space is nothing like the gloomy grime of my youth, and more important, *I* am not a mess. Now in my fifties, I have a wider acceptance of my strengths and weaknesses, my paradoxes, my various natures. I know now that I'm not ever going to become a different person—a person with a spotless, minimalist house, for instance—and I don't care so much. Still, a house, like a soul and a psyche, needs tending to.

When I was a child, my mother would get me to clean my room by playing "Hotel" with me; we'd pretend we were the housekeepers at a hotel, and talk shit about the dirty, entitled guests as we put away my toys. I recall once, at The Blue House, getting dressed up in vintage nightgowns and dusting, like a campy 1960s housewife. Magic and play share the same space in my psyche (and maybe yours?), and just as role-playing inspired me to tidy up in my youth, knowing that cleaning your home can be a ritual often gets me motivated to get my living quarters into shape.

When I was going through my divorce, suddenly the lone tenant in a house that felt too big, still ringing with the bad vibrations of my and my ex's fighting, I knew it had to be cleaned, ritualistically cleaned. But I needed to be cleaned, too! My own vibes were heavy and sad, full of anger and fear. I knew I needed to help myself before I helped my space, lest I just keep smearing the same moody mess all over everything. A bruja friend recommended the services of an *iyabó*, a person in the process of their initiation into the Afro-Caribbean spiritual practice Lucumi, a gorgeous mash-up of traditional African religion and the Catholicism forced upon enslaved people, as well as aspects of practices native to the indigenous people of the Caribbean. The iyabó was an artist named Nova, and for a price I was happy to pay, she created for me two distinct baths, which she had prayed over, and delivered them to my house, twin plastic jugs that once held gallons of crystal-clear water but now swirled with leaves and petals and unknowable grit and oil. She gave me instructions: For one bath, I was to pour the potion over my head while I sat in the tub, letting it splash from my scalp down through my hair, and run down my face and shoulders. I was to sit in the tub and smell the new, sweet smells of the baño, taking handfuls of plant life and using them to scrub my skin, washing away all the old, stagnant energy clogging my psychic pores, all the bad energy projected onto me, all the bad feelings that erupted from my own heart, all of it heavy and heartbreaking. When I was finished, I let the magic water drain from the tub, pulling all those old vibes away. I gathered all the leaves and flowers and threw them in a bag. Then, naked, I stood in the shower and poured the second bath over my head.

Eeeeeeee! It was sort of like a cold plunge, and I did appreciate such a bracing, shocking sensation. Again, I was pleasantly assaulted by gorgeous fragrances. White flower petals stuck to my skin, and tiny leaves and twigs got caught in my hair. I left them there. That was part of the instruction—to not wipe away this purifying baño, but let it dry onto and into me. I took myself to bed and slept naked, the flora scattering in my sheets as I dried. I felt a little like *Snow White*, I'm not going to lie, like some sort of nature princess, not a goddess exactly, but maybe a nymph? Ever was the Goddess here. The beauty and power of her energy and intention swirled through my liquid baños, and I felt incredibly grateful that someone with such a high vibe shared some of her magic with me in this way. I felt truly changed from my bath—not fully healed, of course not, but I felt like I'd pushed through some heavy, energetic obstacle that had been holding me back. I felt freed to move toward a new love. It would take a while to fully slough off the hard shell that had formed around my heart since my divorce, but I felt it cracking.

Next up was a baño for my entire house, now that I myself

felt purified enough to do it. I turned to Nova again, and she made for me two extra-large housecleaning baños, one for my upstairs and one for downstairs. She also gave me a baggie of copal resin harvested from her family's ranch in Mexico, and paper cups of *cascarilla*, ground-up eggshells I was to use as chalk to draw circles around my door, keeping away anyone with ill will.

It felt oddly triumphant to clean my home with Nova's sweet-smelling potions, my windows open to thin the billows of copal streaming from my cauldron. I had come out the other side of a very difficult time, an initiation of sorts, and though at my lowest I could not believe in any goodness life might have in store for me, now, washing and smoking my home, I felt newly baptized and ready for the next suite of ups and downs. I know without a doubt that energy—my energy and the energy of everyone I share my home with—impacts the feeling of this place. It's up to me to keep my own energy well, my psychic immune system healthy, and when things get rough and the vibes sour, to know that this has an impact beyond myself, and to clean accordingly.

A SAINING FOR PETRONILLA

Petronilla de Meath, besides having one of the greatest names in history, also went down in the books for the horrible fact of being the first woman murdered for witchcraft in the very witchy country of Ireland. In the 1300s, Petronilla was the 24-year-old maid who cleaned house, prepped and cooked meals, and overall tidied shit up for Alice Kyteler, a rich lady whose husbands kept dying. When he became sick, husband number 4 voiced a suspicion he was being poisoned by Petronilla and Kyteler, and Kyteler's various stepchildren gathered to accuse her of witchcraft. She was formally accused of such crimes as fashioning potions from unbaptized babies, heading up a coven, and getting it on with an incubus, among other demonic deeds. Petronilla was named as a member of Kyteler's coven and as an accomplice in her crimes. While Kyteler split the scene, never to be seen again, Petronilla was not as privileged, and under torture admitted to assisting her boss in all manners of sorcery, including partaking in a flying ointment.

While light sorcery was almost certainly not in Petronilla's original job description, cleaning the house probably was. In her memory, mingling magic and tidying, I offer this easy way to rid your home of bad-energy bats or whatever unpleasant vibes may be lingering, as well as invite into your living space joy, freshness, and ease.

Saining is a Scots-Irish practice that makes a space sacred, blessing it and protecting it. The primary ingredients are herbs and water, though I like to add a little salt, as I think it is excellent at soaking up yucky energies. For herbs, juniper is best by tradition, and juniper bundles for burning are available at many occult stores. If you happen to live near juniper trees, you can cut some, bind it with natural thread, and hang it upside down to dry. Rosemary and thyme are also powerful purifiers; add some to the juniper for extra oomph. In place of a wand, you may also crumble the dried herbs onto some charcoal in your mini-cauldron. What, you don't have a mini-cauldron? Do you have a birthday coming up, or can you buy yourself a present? I love my mini-cauldron; it's great to have a solidly fireproof container for all the witchy things I like to set on fire. I bet you will love it, too.

For water, your water should be blessed. If you're a legit nature witch and live in close proximity to clear, running natural water, grab some. For the rest of us city folk, filtered water from the front of the refrigerator will have to do. If you happen to be doing your saining on the full moon, leave a jar of water outside with a quartz crystal inside it; I would say such water is blessed. However, if the vibes in your place are bringing you down and you need to sain on the double, do plop a quartz in the water, and say a prayer of intention over it. Talk to the Goddexx or your guides, whomever or whatever you feel has the power to make your water holy. Also, fix a little bowl of salt. Light your herbs. You're ready to sain.

Room by room, move through the space in a clockwise circle. Let the smoke from your herbs reach the corners of each chamber, as well as any little architectural nooks where energy might linger. Dip your fingers in the sacred water and flick it around, in particular getting those corners again. Leave a small pile of salt in each corner. I think it is lovely to speak aloud as you do this, asking all energies that do not serve you, all energies heavy or negative, to leave. If you are saining in the wake of a conflict, ask for that person's energy to return to them. Ask for energy of lightness and joy and whatever represents cozy, sweet home vibes to you to enter your space and bring with it vibes of abundance and serenity. After a day or so, you may sweep up the piles of salt and flush them down the toilet (or scatter them in your stream, you nature witches!).

BESOM BUDDIES

A besom is a classic witch's broom, made of natural materials and still looking more or less like a broom did back in the 1300s. Because they are meant to have a homespun, DIY look to them, this witch craft is actually not too hard, even for folks like me, whose projects eternally retain a preschool aesthetic.

The best thing about making a besom is that you *have* to get into nature. Go where there are trees. Find a big, sturdy stick. It's okay if it's curved or wonky with character. This is your broomstick. Next, you'll need bristles. Hunt about for a whole bunch of long twigs. It's okay if some have leaves or nuts still stuck on them, but you probably should make sure you're not accidentally relocating any insect friends. When you've stuffed your tote with the goods, say thank you to the trees and go home. Make sure you have some twine or cord at home. Lay out a length of cord, lay your bristles about a quarter of the way down it, and get your broomstick nestled in there so that the base is about halfway down your bristle cluster. Got it? Tie that clump of bristles nice and tight. Some witches like to use hot glue, and others like to keep it au natural. As you might imagine, I am pro hot glue, counting among my chosen ancestors many, many drag queens who saw a glue gun as a sacred tool. Use what makes sense to you. Once you get that first cord tied, wrap some additional lengths around your bristles above and below the first one. Once you've got it secure, you can top it off with a more decorative ribbon, hang some precious décor from it, carve a sigil onto the handle, do whatever you like to make it your own. You can also consecrate it, which I very much recommend: pass it through some herbal smoke, spritz it with some crystal or moon water, thank it and ask it to help you keep your home energetically clean.

Your besom won't replace your Swiffer—it likely won't stand up to a real cleaning—but is more like the reiki of brooms, made to gently swish energy out the door.

If you really dig this besom idea but are craft-averse, know that there are many crafty people out there selling their lovely homemade brooms on the internet. There's no shame in patronizing a business witch who has been blessed with DIY talents the Goddexx, in her infinite wisdom, just didn't grant you.

WHEN YOU'RE THE PROBLEM THAT NEEDS A CLEANSE

I recall a shadowy era when, off my meds due to a sudden lack of health care, I started feeling like my home was a little . . .

creepy. Day by day, something just didn't *feel* right. It was very strange—I had always felt such gratitude for living in a big, old house whose vibes were consistently light and airy. What had happened? Did a malignant spirit swoop in? Did a neighbor shoot me the evil eye. Or . . . was it *me?* Yes. Yes, it was. *I* was the source of the bad vibes, not the house I was projecting upon.

In my case (and yours?), I needed to be treating my mental illness. Witchcraft is amazing support, but it does *not* take the place of health insurance and 75 milligrams of Effexor a day. With the help of my support system, I got it sorted out (thanks, Ben!). But my spirit did need cleansing, and, honestly, regular spiritual baths are basic self-care for your psychic immune system. You don't have to wait until you're creeping yourself out to do it!

Here's what I like to use in my own simple baths, but feel free to tweak it according to the season, to what's available to you, and to what you prefer. Just make sure that an ingredient is safe to soak in before you dump it in your tub!

I think salt is the most important ingredient, and probably wouldn't even take a bath if I didn't have a sack of Epsom salts stashed under the sink. Throw a fistful or two in there. You can't go wrong with rosemary and mugwort, and of course flower petals are always lovely. I've put a powerful drip or two of eucalyptus oil into my bath to really feel like I'm steam-cleaning my soul; I've also stuffed cloth tea bags with stinky valerian root and dropped those in when experiencing anxiety, and even filled the tub with ripped-open citrus fruits when needing to rejuvenate my heart. You can make this as fluffy and fussy or as pared-down and practical as you feel like. What's important it to get in the tub, let all the salt and herbs work their magic, and get your head in the right place while you soak and meditate and pray. I always love to go to sleep, preferably naked, right after such a bath, barely drying myself off so that the magic ingredients cling to me as long as possible.

SELL YOUR HOME WITH FOLK CATHOLICISM

I just had to include this popular, if underground (literally!) Catholic spell. Of course, it is not called a *spell*, since Catholics don't *do* spells. It is a . . . what? A prayer? A superstition? Hmmmm. Since no one is at risk of being burned at the stake, I'm going to call a spell a spell and accuse my very own mom, a Catholic lady who once successfully "put a Joseph in the ground," a witch. Which is probably a much more suitable label for her vibe anyway, seeing as she's been excommunicated by the church for remarrying after her divorce, is staunchly pro-choice, and loves her queer daughter. But, anyway. The story goes, my sister was getting married, and my mom, broke as a joke, despaired of not having the funds to help her out with the wedding. At the time, she owned her home in Florida (this was before the subprime mortgage scam took her home, along with so many other people's), and on her property was an extra lot, somewhat small and very jungly. She decided to sell it and use the funds to treat my sister's wedding party to a lovely day-after luncheon. She put the lot on the market, but it didn't sell. And it didn't sell, and it didn't sell. Finally, an aunt who dabbles in the mystical pointed her to a *Joseph in the Ground*, a kit that you can buy to enlist the spiritual powers of Saint Joseph in the selling of real estate.

While you can, like my mom, buy a kit, you can also just get yourself a little statue of Saint Joseph and wrap it lovingly in a cloth to protect it from getting all yucky. Dig a hole near the FOR SALE sign, if there is one, and/or near the street. Pop Joseph in the hole, upside down, facing the property. The kits come with little prayer cards, but you can simply speak out loud to Saint Joseph—who does not look over houses but *does* look over the working class—and ask for his help, thank him for his help, etc. Just be yourself. (That's what so excellent about having an individual magical practice—you can always be yourself, even when you're talking to a deity.)

My mother sold that lot and was able to fete my sister after her big day. After your property sells, get Joe out of the ground, dust him off, and thank him. I'd probably keep him on my altar for a bit, as part of a gratitude practice, and then place him wherever you like.

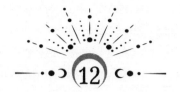

Witch Panic

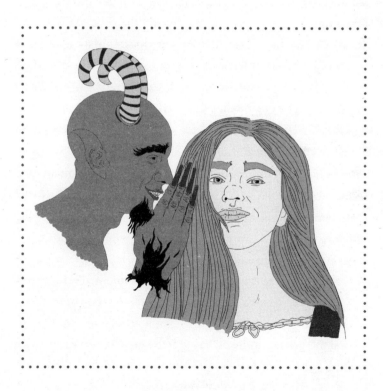

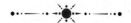

In this book, I've enjoyed highlighting the lives of some witches, both self-proclaimed and accused. For folks who identified and claimed the powerful and always controversial mantle of witch of conjure, like Marie Laveau or Rosaleen Norton, it's easy. These magical individuals were conscious of and open about the way the ephemeral held power in their lives, the intentional ways they engaged with the unknown (and forbidden).

For people like Petronilla de Meath and other victims of witch hysteria, it's a bit more complicated, a bit *both, and.* As in, it's easy to look at these doomed, murdered people, primarily women, and say, "They either were actual witches, or they were the victims of ignorant, superstitious mob mentality." In actuality, I think it is more complex, fraught due to a space-time so hard to comprehend from our present here and now. I think these women (and men) were likely people perhaps a bit more versed in folk arts such as herbs and charms, people who remained more informed by the old ways, who had gut understandings of what we now may be too quick to write off as superstitions. Surely it has already been documented how strong and successful women were often targeted by the witch hunts, as Christianity was policing not only spiritual beliefs but opposition to the patriarchy itself. The witch hunts were charged with making sure individual women did not become too powerful, too autonomous, too wealthy or abundant.

Although I am completely aware that many of the women snagged in the witch hunts and women-hating horrors of history were absolutely *not* witches, even by my rather broad interpretation (an overall *queering* of womanhood, and manhood!), and even though I know many of the murdered had the same hazy or fervent belief in a Christian god as their compatriots, I still choose to claim them as my witchy sisters, and include them in this book. Talking about the ephemeral—magic, energy, vibes, intention, intuition, power—it strikes me as such a blur of reality and fantasy, of play and wish fulfillment. Because I know that there is a metaphysical reality greater than what we see from our spacetime, I am willing to put some stock in it, and this is faith. Because I enjoy the psychological realms of play and power witchcraft conjures, I am willing to accept that at least a portion of it is happy make-believe. This is no less an acceptance of the mystery than the faith part, if you dig. And it is in this sort of mist of belief and imagination that I claim all who died as witches as my ancestors, my coconspirators, no less than any Catholic counts the martyred saints as their religious kin.

And with that, it seems like a good time to get into the history of all this witch hate.

Though I'll be delving into the past, suspicion—or outright hatred—of witches is certainly not a quirk of antiquity. There are so many practioners who feel unsafe being "out" about their spirituality that the funny/not funny phrase "in the broom closet" has become common enough on the internet, describing witches who keep their practices secret from friends, family, and coworkers. Even amid a genuine renaissance of all things witchy, attitudes that range from salacious to ignorant to out-right hateful still exist. Within Christianity, in particular, there seems to be a belief that, unlike other religions that are granted tolerance, witchcraft and paganism are direct affronts; for instance, Christian religious leaders in a county in Texas rallied to shut down a pagan holiday market. Lingering confusion about the differences between witchcraft and Satanism drives much of the insanity, which trickles down from the church into the minds of churchgoers and their children. Young witches report being bullied at school; older witches are threatened with eternal damnation while just trying to live their lives. While in cities the worst blowback might simply be a perennial association with velvet capes, Ren faires, and Dungeons & Dragons that you just don't relate to, the truth is that superstitious fears of (powerful female or empathic male) witches can make a practioner's life very difficult should they live outside centers of diversity and acceptance. In this chapter I'm going to explain the bizarre beginnings of this long-standing witch hate.

Witches have been so famously loathed and scapegoated for so very long, it's easy to forget that it wasn't always that way. Sometime between folk magic being a very normal, ordinary thing and the torture of witches throughout Europe and in the United States, there was a moment in time when even the powerful Catholic Church didn't give too much of a fig about sorcery. It was frowned upon, certainly, but no one was being murdered for it. Perhaps people recalled their mothers and grandmothers whipping up tinctures and following the path of the moon, and so it simply seemed a type of knowledge; female maybe, or from another generation. Perhaps, being older and womanly, its power just wasn't taken seriously. Whatever the reason, it's curious to ponder how Christian Europe went from tolerating vestiges of paganism to murdering so many that one village was said to resemble a burned forest, that many charred funeral pyres stood smoking in the cobbled streets. The answer to what happened—a violent witch paranoia strong enough to continue to mark our own times with prejudice—doesn't fall *completely* on the shoulders of one man, but it sort-of-kind-of *does*: Heinrich Kramer, a Tyrolean inquisitor, obsessive fifteenth-century incel, prototypical troll, and vengeful German churchman who vowed that his humiliating failure to prosecute a badass Austrian party girl would be the last time such a woman escaped his wrath. His work, the *Malleus Maleficarum*, is *the* tract that established witches as the worst of heretics, imagining their lascivious and patently absurd activities, and detailing best practices for proving and punishing their evil.

Let's start at the Catholic Inquisition. Its purpose, when it was founded in the 1100s, was to stomp out heretics—specifically, those working against the Catholic Church, undermining its efforts, making statements about Jesus not being God, and other reasonable, freedom-of-religion observations; many so-called heretics railed against the falseness and hypocrisy of the popes and their riches. The Catholic Church had an if-you're-not-with-us-you're-against-us stance, so to be vocal about finding the Church's teachings fraudulent meant you risked being burned alive as punishment.

At the start of the Inquisition, witchcraft was more of a

secular problem. If you were accused of harassing your neighbor by way of sorcery, you'd wind up before the king's justices, and they handled the matter. The Church wasn't involved in these small-claims-court dustups. But about a hundred years in, Pope Alexander IV suggested that individuals chatting with demons and using sorcery to further their will perhaps *did* equal heresy. The Old Testament was clear about not tolerating spell casters and fortune tellers and those who consult with ghosts; if these activities were ungodly, then they must fall into the realm of the Devil, right? And no one wanted the Church to go belly-up like Lucifer. Under this pope's new conclusion, in the year 1258, it became acceptable for the Inquisition to try individuals for heresy based on an accusation of witchcraft.

Still, that didn't mean that witches were prosecuted for heresy that frequently. The frenzy grew slowly. Famed misogynist Thomas Aquinas fanned the flames, and when the Church turned against its own militia, the Knights Templar, in the 1300s, they used charges of witchcraft to bring them down. When Pope John XXII accused one of his bishops of trying to kill him with sorcery in 1317, it again legitimized the accusation. Then, in the 1340s, Europe was whacked by the plague. And we all know how a pandemic can make people paranoid and prone to conspiracy theories.

Heinrich Kramer was born around 1430, and sources say he was pretty wild about the Church from the get-go. He was young when he joined the Dominicans, the order of monks charged with managing the Inquisition. Heinrich took to it with gusto, and was especially psyched to persecute witches. Now, unfortunately for him, though there were theoretical grounds to prosecute witches for heresy, Heinrich found it hard to get a witch before the Inquisition's assessors. I guess that, just like today, the medieval period had some folks who trended toward decency and chillness, while others, like Heinrich, veered toward unhinged drama. He had a particularly tough time making a case against a Tyrolean woman named Helena Scheuberin, in the town of Innsbruck, situated in a snow-y, lake-y region that encompasses northern Italy and eastern Austria.

Helena seems pretty cool. Hans P. Broedel, in his book *The Malleus Maleficarum and the Construction of Witchcraft*, describes her as an "aggressive, independent woman not afraid to speak her mind." But she found herself on the receiving end of some town gossip after a noble knight named Jörg Speiss turned up dead. Before he died, while seeking medical help, he was warned by his doctor to avoid the home of Helena Scheuberin.

Helena had a rich husband. Maybe they threw big parties, maybe they were doing opium or drinking beer brewed with belladonna, maybe Noble Knight Jörg was hitting the medieval intoxicants too hard at Helena's ragers and the doctor knew it—maybe that's what he meant. I mean, I'm deeply speculating here. But it is weird that the doctor was literally, "Keep away from Helena's house or you'll die." And then he died. Was he having an affair with her, and was he poisoned by her jealous husband? Maybe he had some sort of dirt on Helena and *she* was poisoning him? Do I watch too much *ID Discovery*? Word on the streets of Innsbruck was that it *might* have been witchcraft.

This was the kind of tea Heinrich lived for. Word of this

mysterious death, the doctor's ominous warning, Helena's "aggressive and independent" personality, the townspeople's gossip of magic—it sends him flying to Innsbruck faster than a colonial witch with a broom up her vagina. He set himself up with some sermons at the local church and gets to harassing his target. But good luck, Heinrich, because the lass lives up to her fearsome reputation. Upon meeting her assessor in the street, Helena jumped in his face, shouting, "Fie on you, you bad monk, may the falling evil take you!" Let's hear that again: *Fie on you. You bad monk. May the falling evil take you.* I have chills. This is an amazing diss. She's good.

Helena mostly avoids Heinrich's sermons, *of course*, and urges others to as well, and Heinrich takes this as evidence of her sorcery. You would think he'd be happy about her absence, since when she *does* attend church she heckles him, calling him an "evil man in league with the Devil." Yes, Helena, flip that script!

Heinrich eventually managed to begin a trial for Helena, along with some other women, her witchy girl gang no doubt. But the local authorities weren't having it. Maybe they're Team Helena, maybe they don't believe in witchcraft. Maybe they think Heinrich is a nerd, or that the Catholic Church is a bully. Either way, the powers of Innsbruck actually kick Heinrich out of town. I can and will imagine the victory bash Helena and her rich hubby threw when that happened. Let the nightshade-laced mead flow! But a troll doesn't give up that easily. Heinrich was far from done with Helena and the witches of Innsbruck. In a big baby move, he went straight to the Vatican and whined to the pope about how terribly he was treated in Tyrol, basically asking him to write a note telling everyone they have to take his authority seriously.

Pope Innocent VIII—wait, can you even with these popes? That name is so ironic it's actually offensive. Pope Innocent VIII invested in the trade of enslaved Africans, he ran a scheme targeting noblewomen and accusing them of heresy so the Church could seize their money, *and he literally* created positions within the Church to be sold to the highest bidder. And he names himself "Innocent," like he's a zero-calorie can of Le Croix. Anyway, Pope Innocent does oblige Heinrich—he'd recently promoted the troll to Head of the Inquisition, and they were buds. The pope drew up a papal decree called the *Summis Desiderantes Affectibus*, which is Latin for "you better be nice to Heinrich." It affirms that witches are *real*, that they are *heretics*, that the Church has the right to try them, and that anyone who interferes are themselves heretics and subject to punishment.

Heinrich returned to Innsbruck, all smug with his papal decree. Let's take a moment to envision this jerk, with the help of some existing medieval portraits. Medieval artists had an infamously strange gaze. In some paintings, Heinrich's face appears to be a popped football, his bald head ringed with a classic Dominican fringe. One portrait depicts him as emaciated with a prominent chin wattle; in another he's plump, his eyes quite near his nose. One portrait is not so odd. His bulky, black jacket looks cozy, and is stylishly belted. He sports a little beret, and his cheekbones look like the fruits of a YouTube contouring tutorial. Willem Dafoe could convincingly play him in a biopic. He's seated in a little wooden room, caught up in his thoughts, lost in a reverie. He looks like a poet being gently touched by the muse, not like a medieval serial killer penning his macabre how-to book.

Okay, now that we're all imagining Willem Dafoe striding into a medieval village, waving a papal bull, let's continue. With the legitimizing Church document in hand, the leaders of Innsbruck had less power to evict Heinrich from the village. A witch trial against Helena Scheuberin and her best bitches officially commenced. The trial lasted about a month, from Leo season in the summer to Virgo season at the start of fall. What's interesting is, though there were townspeople accusing Helena and company of witchcraft, none of them made mention of the Devil. It was the Church that was equating witchcraft—pagan folk magic—with Satanism, and Heinrich did bring forth accusations of fraternizing with the Devil, celebrating the orgiastic witches' sabbath, and all that. Apparently, Heinrich based much of his accusation against Helena on her supposed promiscuity. But in spite of these efforts, the trial ended without a confession. There was a month or so of respite; Heinrich left town, Helena returned to her sumptuous home and partied, or recuperated. But after not so long, Heinrich was back. He would get a confession from his witch, if he had to torture it out of her. Which, as we know, was the Church's favorite method of extracting confessions for crimes that didn't actually exist.

Like the trial, the torturing of Helena and the other accused women lasted about a month. A popular medieval device for such occasions was a hideous contraption called the *strappado*. A person's hands were tied behind their back, and then they were lifted high into the air, so that their body hung heavily, contorted, and their shoulders dislocated as they dangled. Weights were sometimes attached to the body, to make an impossibly gruesome situation more so. The victim would generally die within an hour.

There were other methods of getting women to confess to nonexistent love affairs with Satan. Sleep deprivation often brought about a successful disclosure; after being kept awake by Devil-obsessed maniacs for four or five consecutive nights, who wouldn't start hallucinating they were the consort of the Horned God?

One of Heinrich's favorite torture tasks was to have an accused witch carry a chunk of red-hot iron for precisely three steps, without dropping it. If you could do this, you were *not* a witch, even though it seems that it would take supernatural powers to override your body's instinct to toss it from your swiftly blistering hands. If you *did* have a natural reaction, if you burst into tears and screamed "Fuck!" and dropped the glowing blob of iron to the ground, you *were* a witch.

A final common torture for the era was the "swimming" of witches, that famous lose-lose in which the accused was hogtied and dropped into water. If she lived, she was a witch, and was imminently doused in flames. If she drowned, well, the poor lass had been innocent after all, but she's gone to a better place now, hasn't she? Actually, in this case, maybe?

I couldn't find any writings that specified which malevolent method Heinrich employed to manifest a confession from Helena, but a month of torture probably featured a sickening variety. However, at the end of it all, Heinrich *lost*. The Church could not prove that Helena Scheuberin had murdered the noble knight Jörg Spiess with witchcraft or otherwise. Helena was truly unbreakable; whatever torture was deployed upon her, she did not crack, and I'd like to imagine the barrage of insults she hurled upon the weaselly inquisitor.

Heinrich, as you can tell, was not the sort to adopt a "you win some, you lose some" attitude about his witch trials. He had a hard time letting go. His obsession with Helena continued to fester, and he stayed in Innsbruck to harass her, even after the local authorities again demanded he leave. It took an appeal to the bishop to finally get him to quit bothering the woman, and depart Innsbruck. Heinrich gathered up all of his fury and resentment, his wounded Dominican ego and Catholic righteousness, and crawled back under a rock in Cologne, Germany. He focused the storm of psychedelic rage swirling inside him, and he began to write.

Published in 1486, the *Malleus Maleficarum* was Heinrich Kramer's life work, his lasting legacy. Although fellow Dominican Jacob Sprenger was listed as a coauthor on editions published after 1519, Heinrich died in 1505, and scholars now credit the entire authorship of the *Malleus Maleficarum* to Heinrich. There's also an internet rumor that Sprenger fucking *hated* Kramer, but I couldn't find anything to really back that up.

So, what's the *Malleus*, this medieval piece of revenge porn penned by a fifteenth-century incel, actually about? Heinrich meant it to be the legal bones behind the Christian scripture, "Thou shalt not suffer a sorceress to live." First and foremost, it's a legal document; it includes and elaborates upon Pope Innocent's papal bull instituting witchcraft as heresy; it lobbies the courts of Europe to prosecute it as such. It delineates a sort of *best practices* for trying witches, advising that judges wear a charm of blessed salt around their neck, that witches should be stripped and shaved and led into the courtroom backwards. It explained how to gain confessions via torture and the sort of punishment by death to pursue once witchery has been established. As burning at the stake was the most traditional way to dispose of heretics in general, it was easily applied to witches. Heinrich believed God would not allow an innocent person to be mistakenly murdered for witchcraft, so that took care of any concern about wrongful death and what have you.

Now, officially establishing witchcraft as heresy effectively created another legal rule: it became mandatory that everyone *believe* in witches and witchcraft, as defined by the Church; to deny their evil legitimacy would subject you to their fate. If you perhaps *wanted* to believe in witches but worried that you just didn't know enough about them or really understand their customs, here's where Heinrich really shines—in the portion of the *Malleus* that describes what exactly the witches are up to. I think their most interesting recorded activity was causing the penises of men to vanish from their bodies and reappear up high in the treetops, cozied together in a nest, as if they were a flock of baby birds; and like a flock of baby birds, the witches would feed these magically castrated phalluses a meal of oats. Don't believe me? I don't blame you. But, let me quote from the book: "What are we to think about those witches who shut up penises in what are sometimes prolific numbers, twenty or thirty at a single time, in a bird's nest or some kind of box, where they move about in order to eat oats and fodder, as though they were alive—something which many people have seen and is reported by common gossip?" *Many people* saw this? Like, *many?* Okay. I mean, common gossip is never wrong.

Now, to Heinrich's credit, he didn't think that the witches were actually stealing penises from the bodies of men. He wasn't *crazy.* To remove a penis you'd need a proper demon's help, and, frankly, most witches weren't that powerful. What they could do is make you hallucinate that your penis had vanished, and then give you a vision of it eating oats in a tree. Likewise, the witches of medieval Europe couldn't actually turn you into an animal, because they didn't have that level of demonic power. They could only make you *think* they'd turned you into an animal.

Props to Heinrich for simultaneously minimizing the witches' powers while affirming their terror and malevolence. Hallucination or no, who wants to look down and find their junk no longer in their pants? Not I. And remember, lest you scoff at this tale and call it unbelievable, you now risk being accused of heresy yourself.

The *Malleus* goes on to relay much delicious witchy doings, such as the tale of a woman who, miffed that she had not been invited to a wedding, flew to a hillside, pissed into a bowl, stirred her urine counterclockwise, and brought down a storm upon the festivities. A great spell to try yourself next time you're feeling left out of your community.

Actually, in case you *are* interested, here's what you need to do to become a medieval-style witch. Much of this lore had already been established by the Catholic Church by the time Heinrich came along, but he elaborated upon and popularized it. First, you must swear off Christianity and enter into a pact with the Devil. Check. Next, you put your money where your mouth is and seal the deal by actually having sex with the Devil. Now, the Devil, being Satanic, has particular tastes. While he was reportedly a good time in the sack—a seductive lover and all that—he also required his new acolytes to prove their love with the "osculum infame." Also called "the shameful kiss," it was but a kiss upon the Devil's anus, or a bit of a medieval rim job, depending upon the enthusiasm of the witch.

The Devil would then show his appreciation by granting the witch the gift of flight, very important if she was to make it to the frequent witch gatherings in the deepest woods, presided over by Satan himself. Who'd want to miss that?! By taking a special ointment made from the fat of unbaptized babies and applying it to a broom or household chair, the objects would then be enchanted enough to serve as a vehicle to get you to the deep-woods witch party. (Of course, there are theories that the ointments were made with hallucinogens, not baby fat, and then inserted into the vagina via broomstick or chair leg, causing quite a "flight.")

While this was all standard Church lore, Heinrich claimed that if a witch for some reason was unable to journey to the Satanic Rave, maybe because she was lazy, or suffered social anxiety or was under a seven-day quarantine for Covid, she could join remotely, by lying on her left side and breathing a blue vapor from her mouth. The vapor acted as a sort of medieval zoom room, allowing the witch to observe the goings-on from the comfort of her cottage. But really, you'd rather be there in person, as the gatherings were veritable sex parties, and possibly the only place a lady could get it on with a demon. Strangely, Heinrich noted the "nobility" of the demons' natures, and suggested that many of them probably didn't even *want* to have sex with the witches; they were just doing it because it was, like, their job. It feels a little like Heinrich is projecting right here. Obviously, demons *love* having sex with witches. After the orgy portion of the gathering is over, everyone gets to cursing and hexing, and the slaughtering and eating of unbaptized babies. Or, the drinking of. After they've been slow-cooking in the cauldron all this time, the flesh falls off the bones, creating a rather slurpable bone broth. Don't you dare *yuck* at me—I'm simply sharing the knowledge of a rather important Dominican monk, okay? If you want to see for yourself, there is currently a first edition of *Malleus* for sale on the internet for $202,000.

While the *Malleus* has obviously stood the test of time—here we are, talking about it—it had a bit of a rough start. The top theologians of the day, while clearly not averse to burning your average heretic alive, drew the line at witch hunts. Heinrich went out trying to get some Catholic influencers, some folks over at the University of Cologne, to blurb his little book, and he was told that what he'd written was unethical, illegal, and also inconsistent with established Catholic beliefs on demonology.

So, Heinrich does what I, as an author, have always wished I could do—he just makes up some praise for his work and forges a celeb signature or two. But Heinrich did find a lot of support among his fellow Dominicans. As the prime movers of the Inquisition, in addition to fighting heresy, they'd taken up arms against prostitution and sodomy (wouldn't you know, a lot of people who don't like witches even today also don't like queers and sex workers), and the Dominicans loved the *Malleus Maleficarum*. With their endorsement, boom, the book starts flying off the shelves, and Heinrich is a celeb. If you need a talking head for your anti-witchcraft lecture series, or an expert witness at your village witch trial, he's your man. He's in high demand all over Europe, and he even receives a patronage from the Patriarch of Venice. And he's prolific; like the Joyce Carol Oates of anti-witchcraft propaganda, he's always got a new discourse or sermon or defense to promote. Heinrich is made Papal Nuncio, a sort of diplomat to the pope, and his inquisition terrain grows to include the Czech Republic. He's failing up. While there were always some within the church who thought Heinrich was a ding-dong, the secular world and its justice systems would rely on the *Malleus* throughout the Renaissance.

From 1484 to 1750, about 200,000 people were accused of witchcraft, and were tortured and/or killed in Western Europe. Famously, most were women—about three quarters of those charged. The *Malleus,* of course, explained this tendency for women to fall under the thrall of Satan—their inherent weak faith and sexed-up carnality made them easy marks. "They are defective in all the powers of both soul and body," Heinrich wrote, doubling down with the statement, "woman, therefore, is evil as a result of nature." A man would, on occasion, fall prey to the lure of witchcraft, but it was usually in a more macho, power-seeking way, not as a result of an interior weakness.

There was a hierarchy of evil types of women—sexy concubines were the *worst,* followed by midwives, with their ancient knowledge and access to babies, and lastly, women who dominated their husbands. But no matter if you didn't see yourself represented here—the *Malleus* claimed that *any* woman would likely find herself "succumbing to her passions and becoming a witch." Truly the only way to ensure that you didn't find yourself with your face planted in the Devil's buttocks was to live in a religious retreat, having taken a vow of devout chastity. And so we see the virgin versus whore dichotomy dressed up as nun versus witch. Though this was the only foolproof way to prevent your weak, female nature from sliding into witchcraft, Heinrich also understood that most people were unlikely to thrive in such an extreme environment; only a certain type of femme would be able to stand it. The rest, he claimed, "are doomed to become witches, who cannot be redeemed; and the only recourse open to the authorities is to ferret out and exterminate all witches." As Heinrich delved deeper into his obsession, it became increasingly clear that "witches" was simply a code name for "women."

Heinrich died in 1505, leaving the party while he was still

having fun. For 200 years after his death, the *Malleus* reigned, outselling even the Bible. His legacy traveled across the Atlantic with the European colonizers bound for North America, and laid the groundwork for the eventual hanging of witches in what's now Salem, Massachusetts. In 1684, Increase Mather, president of Harvard University, gave the *Malleus* a shout-out in his incredibly titled work, *An essay for the recording of illustrious providences wherein an account is given of many remarkable and very memorable events, which have happened this last age, especially in New-England. By Increase Mather, Teacher of a Church at Boston in New-England.* Mather's text reads like the script of a Blumhouse movie, with flying hammers, Satan taking the form of deer and crows, sulfurous smells, frying pans hanging inside chimneys, and the inhabitants of many houses generally molested by demons.

Thank you for sticking with me through this disturbing yet informative history of witch hate and general misogyny. If you are a witchy person, but you're a little scared to explore further, this might be the reason. If you are a witch, but you keep it in the broom closet, you can trace your fears and the fear of those around you back to this one little man hundreds of years ago, who could never get over one Helena Scheuberin. Seeing how witches are thriving today in the midst of what feels like a renaissance, I almost feel bad for the schmuck, and thought briefly of lighting a candle for him on my altar that he find his way from human spacetime forevermore. Then I thought, *Fie on you, you bad monk! May the falling evil take you!* And I lit one for Helena instead.

A PROTECTION PARTY IN HONOR OF HELENA SCHEUBERIN

What is a party if not a group ritual? With this spell, you're asked to make the subtext the plot, and invite your nearest and dearest over with the intent to participate in a ritual shaped like a party. The purpose: to raise protective joy for all participants as well as all the world's peoples vulnerable to the violent scapegoating of the ignorant.

Be overt in your invitation, and invite only people you believe will embrace such an event; you don't want skeptical bad vibes weighing down your energy. Let people know they will be expected to eat, drink, laugh, dance, and be merry with the intention of raising holy, protective joy. Have guests check with you before bringing along a friend; I'm not much of a control freak, but you do want to have a sense of whom you're making magick with.

The day of the rager, give your home—or wherever you'll be partying—a spiritual cleanse. Speak aloud to the spirits and let them know what's happening; request their blessing and support. Fashion an altar especially for this ritual. Protective crystals like amethyst, selenite, quartz, and obsidian, all black-colored stones, are fantastic for power and protection. For joy, I like red stones: carnelian, red jasper, strawberry and crimson quartz, as well as citrine, lapis, rose quartz, and pyrite. Black candles are excellent for protection, and I like pink, orange, red, and yellow candles for joy. Of course, if you have colors or stones you associate with either protection or joy, use them! You might also want to have on your altar images of particular ancestors or deities you wish to invoke; and you might want to invite your guests to bring something to contribute to the altar.

Herbs that are traditionally linked to protection include rosemary, sage, basil, lavender, echinacea, and peppermint; utilize them for their smoke and/or scent via the herbs themselves, candles, or oils. Lavender, basil, and rosemary *also* do double duty as supporters of joy, like their joyful fellow herbs chamomile, lemon balm, ginger, chives, and dandelion. Work with these herbs and their properties while conjuring your party menu. Chive dip? Classic. If dandelions are blooming, make the blossoms into fritters. Ginger punch. Lemon balm sorbet. Chamomile donuts. Roast some party nuts with salt and rosemary (or with honey and lavender!). A caprese salad with fresh basil. A candy dish of Peppermint Patties. Some hot echinacea tea to end the night. There are an endless number of both herbs and recipes for you to play with; what is most important is not to overextend yourself. Keep it manageable, so that it can be enjoyable and you are able to focus ritual intention into every snack or beverage you prepare. When you set out your food and make that little tag letting folks know its gluten-free or has dairy, also note its magical intention, so that your guests may bring their focus to it as they indulge.

Dancing is a great way to raise energy. Be intentional by making a playlist beforehand, keeping an ear out for songs that affirm the power of joy, as well as songs that affirm the power of self-worth and self-protection—and community worth and community protection.

Give yourself a moment to center and pray or spellcast about twenty minutes before your guests show up. Depending on how bold or shy you feel, you may want to lead your friends in a simple intention, meditation, circle-casting, spell, or blessing at some point in the night; conversely, you might just want to let the party ritual take its own shape and direction, knowing that once the guests have arrived, the beats are thumping, and the food is flowing that the ritual is in full swing and, to some extent, your work is done (until the cleanup starts).

LAURIE'S EGG OF LIGHT

Once, on a performance tour with the author Laurie Weeks, I became accustomed to her shouting, "Egg of light! Egg of light!" whenever she perceived herself, or our tour as a whole, to be in a precarious circumstance. The year was 1999, and we were two vanfuls of queer, trans, and feminist misfit spoken-word artists traversing the United States; actions as simple as entering a restroom or filling up the gas tanks frequently had an edge of danger. "Egg of light!" Laurie would holler in her adorable, raspy voice, and we would imagine all of it—our vans, ourselves, one another—ensconced in a warm and protective egg of light.

This is one of those great practices/spells you can do on the spot, whenever you find yourself in a threatening situation, be that threat social, physical, imaginary, who cares. Sometimes you just feel like you need that Egg of Light, and it is eternal and nonjudgmental—it is always there for you! However, before you start using it on the spot, I think it's great to do a larger Egg of Light meditation at home, to really familiarize yourself with what the egg feels like, looks like, seems like to you. You might even want to make this a regular sort of practice/spell/meditation, so that you become accustomed to the egg's protective glow. This might help you both need it less often and be able to summon it more quickly and powerfully when you do.

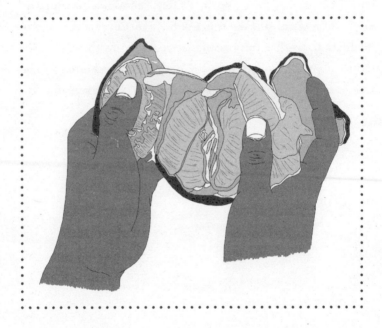

Bring Me Love, and Sex. And Love.

I 've saved this chapter—love—for last, because it's the best, and it's the worst. It's certainly the number one reason people reach out for magic, to bring love into their lives or to help them heal from a breakup (or enact revenge if things went south in a particularly crummy way). There is *so much out there* regarding love spells that I really want to be saying something different here. Not just for the creative challenge, but because I think we need new approaches to love, and magic—being a sort of rogue and defiant tradition that embraces experimentation— seems very well-suited to help us with a relational overhaul.

Why do I think we need new approaches to romance? Well, hit shuffle on your music library, and chances are it lands on a

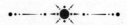

song bemoaning the uniquely particular agony of love. Watch a movie, read a book, binge a show, there it is. Is romantic love just *inherently painful*, prone to disaster? Or is it us—our muddy psyches, the expectations we bring—that leave us sobbing in the shower?

We all live in a culture that prioritizes romantic dyads. It's *literally* all we see. Chances are, we were raised in a dyad, by people raised in a dyad, everyone feeding on media and assorted cultural offerings that insist on the primacy of the dyad. The one-two punch of the dyad is 1. It's the *only* type of relationship; and 2. You *must be* in a relationship that sets us all up to look for that fairy-tale perfect person. The soulmate. This puts a lot of pressure on you, whoever you're hooking up with.

What would it be like if our cultures and families didn't encourage us to partner up? What if living single was known to be as rich and meaningful as being in a partnership? What if having multiple relationships, serious or casual or a mixture of both, were the norm? I could imagine that those synced to our culture's current mode—a person looking for one other person to be their everything—would seem a bit wild: unimaginative, claustrophobic, obsessive. And surely many dyadic relationships play out that way! Partners have to put in effort to keep the excitement alive in a dyad—lesbian bed death is *not* just for lesbians. They have to remember to take space for themselves, to not become codependent.

I'm not a person who decries monogamy as *less evolved* or any of that crap. What I'm talking about here is really a thought experiment. We don't know what this dream society would look like, what unique heartbreaks, habits, expectations, and mind fucks would plague its lovers. It is really possible that the human heart is just a beating box of problems, and that romance in any configuration will bring along its own slew of issues. There is, of course, a spiritual way to look at this: that love is one of the most powerful teachers of life lessons. And if we believe that we're "here," wherever this is, at least in part to help our spirits evolve, surely loving other humans, the joy and pain of it, is a formidable instructor.

I remember being very young and becoming obsessed with the glamour of romance as seen on TV. *Happy Days, Laverne & Shirley, The Facts of Life, The Brady Bunch*—the shows of my childhood *did* have storylines other than romance, but who cares? Romance was primary and crucial. I wondered what it would be like to fall enormously in love, the way cartoon femmes in Disney stories fell in love. I wanted to swoon and be transported. I wanted it to change me from this thing I was into a whole new, more glittering thing.

As my home life became increasingly stressful, the promise of romance became an easy escape to indulge. It was *everywhere*, and it was acceptable for a girl to be a little *boy crazy*. It didn't matter if my parents fought or if my stepfather was an alcoholic, if my birth father had peaced out or if the kids at my Catholic school thought I was a weirdo—this kid life was meaningless, a holding pen. Eventually I would grow up and *fall in love*, and then my real life would begin. The thrill of love would be all that mattered, would make up for all the bullshit. I would confide to my *soulmate* all I'd endured, and he (of course a he, duh) would pet my head and say shit like, "Now, now, my darling, those days are over. It's just love and support for you from here on out." If it sounds like what I was imagining was, um, *a daddy*, you wouldn't be totally wrong. But as I laid in my teenage bed, getting high off the array of heartthrobs I'd papered my walls with—a pouting George Michael morphing into a shirtless Billy Idol morphing into any number of goth rockers on the sulky-to-menacing spectrum—concepts like *daddy issues, attachment styles, love language,* and *love addict* were still decades away.

I got sober in the midst of a long-term relationship that was exciting and lovely in some ways, and in others, plain miserable. I hadn't thought my partner was anything like my moody, avoidant, alcoholic dad—he was a young trans guy, so how could he resemble that Polish, depressive cis straight guy even a little? And yet, I've learned that I love a sulky man with control issues and some substance abuse history. Getting sober was like switching the lights on in a hoarder's basement of feelings, seeing all the messes I hadn't let go of yet or hadn't looked at head-on. In there, like a creepy, broken doll, was little me, still waiting for my prince to come. The tumultuous relationship I was in would not survive my sobriety, and in the process, I'd learned many hard truths about love. The phrase *inner child* hadn't yet been reclaimed by younger generations, and was far too cringey of a concept for me right then, but it really was a reckoning with that small, hurt part of myself. Together we mourned the ways we hadn't been loved right, understanding that the love we craved from partners was meant to come to us from parents. We'd never get it from a lover; it just wasn't appropriate. The best I could do was love that needy little part of myself, and hope to get my head on straight about romance and relationships.

I think I've tried nearly everything. I've both been non-monogamous and simply dating; I've been married and open; I've been slutty and discerning. I've *tried* to be solo poly, but old systems are hard to rewire, and I capitulate to the romance of *being wifed*. Currently, I'm as traditional as they come—queerly married, a mom, pretty monogamish but maybe some wiggle room if I'm traveling, or run into Matt Dillon. My attraction to people with the same essential profile as my birth father—depressive, a bit stern—has not waned, though insisting on additional qualities (medication, therapized, self-aware) make a difference.

When we do a love spell, it is, in a sense, the best of us—the sweetest, most hopeful, optimistic, and loving part of our psyche opening up. It's very vulnerable. We put our energy out there, and love comes to us. People are drawn in—messy people with scars and backpacks of drama. There's no way for it not to get messy. You can't make space for love without risking hurt. So, before you sit down at your altar with your list of love demands, it's best to do some hardcore thinking about where you're coming from, and what you're bringing with you. Have you considered . . .

Your family of origin? What did you learn about love from watching the people who raised you? What unspoken rules were inferred? What did you internalize? What were you taught that love—and a lover, a relationship—would be for you? What type of lover or relationship were you expected to want? What sort of person imprinted upon you as a *love object*?

Attachment style? This psychological theory of how and why we bond with boos the way we do comes from the early 1990s, but you probably know about it from the internet. The core thought is, based on conclusions you came to *as an infant*, informed by the way you were cared for, you tend to relate to your love object in a manner that is either anxious, avoidant, disorganized, or secure. Anxious: codependent tendencies, boundaries are scary, afraid to burden their relationships with their needs. Avoidant: shuts down and pulls away, maniacally independent, can't handle a partner's humanity. Disorganized: super checked-out, unable to empathize, great at sabotage. Secure, obviously, is where we all want to be: these unicorns are able to validate their needs and expect them to be met, neither hiding nor people pleasing, just simply existing in their truths, radiating kindness. Sounds nice. Congratulations to the one percent of humanity that does *not* relate to Philip Larkin's famous poem, "This Be the Verse": *They fuck you up, your mum and dad. / They may not mean to, but they do.* As for the rest of us, we'll spend our twenties in and out of dramatically shitty relationships, climb wearily into our thirties determined to figure out what the *fuck* is wrong with us, then spend the rest of our lives putting what we discovered into practice. And it *does* work—all the effort I've put in to challenge my worst presumptions about romance, to get mentally healthy and chemically balanced, to value and trust myself—it all results in better partnerships. And it's not just because like attracts like, and now I'm swiping on some holier, white-light dating app. It's more that, when something feels bad, I'm more likely to leave. And *that* is everything.

Now, if you've made it through this rather heavy essay about love and *still* want to cast some spells, I've got one for whatever sort of love or lust you're after.

ZIZILIA SEX SPELL

Zizilia is an *alleged* goddess in the ancient Polish pantheon, which I sort of love. To be an *alleged* goddess! It makes me think of Pluto, tossed out of the solar system but forever in our hearts and psyches as astrological ruler of the underworld. Zizilia, as a goddess who rules sexuality, has some things in common with Pluto, who represents our shadow selves and darker desires: fear and depth. While Zizilia also rules sex-adjacent realms such as love, motherhood, childbirth, and marriage, it's her *Holy Slut* aspect I'd like to address here, to help you get the kind of sex you want to have.

In order to get the kind of sex you want to have, the first thing you must do is *know* what kind of sex you want to be having. What do you want it to look like, feel like? What's the vibe? What sort of person would you like to be having it with—what gender, what aesthetic? What do you want to *happen*? Are there toys, accessories? Are their costumes, roles, certain words? Write about it, all of it, in a journal or notebook. Dare to be completely honest with yourself. No sexual partner is ever going to read your mind. Be as clear as possible, so that when Zizilia arranges for you to meet your dream lover, you have the ability to clearly ask for what you want. Take your finished pages and bury them in the earth. (Make sure there is no identifying information on the pages, that it is totally anonymous. The Universe knows you, no need to state your name!) A Monday would be astrologically good, as Mondays are holy to the moon, where so much of our desire lives; or Friday, dedicated to Venus, which determines our sexual aesthetic.

While you wait for your amour to appear, keep the spell going with lemon balm, a sexy herb that ups your capacity for desire physically and magically. Drink lemon balm tea, put leaves of fresh lemon balm in your undies (this from an olde folke magick custom of maidens placing lemon balm leaves in the "mouth of a beehive," *wink*), carry dried or fresh lemon balm in a red bag somewhere on you, place lemon balm under your pillow at night. After your spell has come to fruition, and you've had some next-level sex, it might be polite to burn a candle for Zizilia as a thank you.

BRING ME LOVE BLOOD (ORANGE) BATH

I recently learned, from a Vedic astrologer friend, that my aversion to details is quite deep, knitted into my astrological makeup. Details, said my friend, block inspiration and prevent the Universe from bringing me gifts. I have always, always, *always* felt this! In fact, once, in my early twenties, while in San

CC••·—·· 236 ··—··•CC

Francisco, I was pining for love and thinking about a particular love spell where you write down exactly all the qualities you look for in a lover and burn a candle about it. This is, actually, a pretty powerful spell, and it works. For some people. I found myself struggling with it right away. Trying to Frankenstein myself my own perfect lover swiftly felt creepy, and limiting! Why rely on my feeble imagination, my limited life experience? What I wanted, really, was to be wowed by love, to experience the surprise of another human being. It wasn't, I realized, about the Universe catering to my preferences; it was about *me* being open to the various forms love can take, and not allowing what I *think* are my preferences (but are maybe just brainwashing/habit/control) to dictate the way love enters my life.

I decided that what I would do is simply call *love* into my days. Love the energy, the concept, the vibration, the deity, the experience—what is it, even? I didn't pretend to know. Right then and there, still newly queer, having just followed a low-key sociopath across the country only to be left for the most boring dude in the world, and *then* having landed in a neighborhood of feral dykes with pierced faces and shaved heads who liked to mosh on the dance floor and spank each other at the bar— well, my head was *spinning*. Clearly, I knew nothing about love, lust, the possibilities of relationships. Why give the Universe my dinky, low-ball Christmas list? No. *Just bring me love. And sex. And love. Help me to know it.* That's what I said—and I said it out loud, even though my roommates, total squares, were home and probably thought I was nuttier than they'd surmised.

So. The bathtub will be your altar. I sure hope you have a bathtub. If you don't, use your shower. Into your bathtub, bring a few blood oranges. I selected blood oranges because they seemed extra passionate, extra deep and mysterious, like sex and love. And oranges, "golden apples," are sacred to Aphrodite, the Greek goddess of love, as well as Oshun, the Yoruba goddess of love. Oshun also loves cinnamon, so bring some cinnamon sticks with you as well. Roses are iconic when it comes to love, so red rose petals are welcome, as are red and orange candles.

Once in the bath, tear the oranges open with your fingers. It can be messy; it should be messy! Let the juice and the pulp fall onto you and into the water. (If you are showering, be beneath the spray, and rub the fruit and the cinnamon onto your body.) Swish your bathwater around you and then lean back and meditate. *Bring me love . . . Just bring me love. And sex. And love. Help me to know it.* Let these simple statements swirl around your head; speak them out loud, in whispers or hollers. Be still within your bath, feeling your own vibrations and the vibrations of everything around you. Possibly all of it is love. Masturbate if you feel like it. You already are love, and sex, but such alchemy occurs when two (or more) bodies made of sex and love come together to see what it's all about. You already know at least half of it.

When you're done with your bath (or shower), come out of the tub but don't towel off. Allow yourself to air dry. Hopefully you'll catch a whiff of citrus or spice on your skin. I like to do this spell before bed, and sleep naked if possible. Be sure to record your dreams in the morning. Feel free to save an orange peel or cinnamon stick from the ritual, keeping it on your altar or tucked into your pocket.

BEYOND THE PHYSICAL THIRD EYE SPELL

This is a spell for anyone who feels trapped by the limitations of their *type*. Maybe you have recognized that your *type* is actually people who aren't very nice, or good to you. Maybe you are realizing you have looks-ist biases against certain people, and you don't want your love life to be ruled by surface considerations. We know there are more to humans than what we see, and part of love is getting to go deep with another. How sad it is that we limit ourselves by what our culture has convinced us is "hot."

Maybe you are already with someone, and you're finding there is something about them that annoys you—a little something, a petty something. The kind of shit that should not interfere with something as noble and good as *love*. But we are glorified monkeys. Sometimes (frequently) we are petty and narrow. Two things that do not mesh well with love.

If this stings, do not fear. Your third eye's got you. Located between your eyebrows, this swirling energy center was first discovered by Indian mystics a very, very long time ago, but maybe you have felt yours as recently as today? I often feel a slight tickle, or vibration, at that spot, and have found that if you sit in meditation, focusing on it, it often makes itself known to you.

The third eye is perhaps the seat of our highest self. It contains our spiritual, mystical, intuitive potential. It is the seat of whatever psychic powers we might develop. It is our connection to higher consciousness, and it's where we can turn when we want to upgrade what it is we are attracted to. It is the point on our energetic body that is going beyond the physical, the material world with all its illusions and delusions. The third eye can help us home in on who has the right *energy* for us to partner with.

Sexual attraction is *real*, and powerful. It's also much more malleable, mutable, than we realize. And it's *also* subject to lots and lots of brainwashing from the dominant culture, which would have us believing only skinny, cisgendered white or "exotic" (read: brown people fetishized for white consumption) people are lovable. The *actual* world, and our actual lives, show us the lie of that every day, but we are still bombarded. And it is nice to lean into the third eye for support, and to support its powers in turn.

The candle colors for this are shades of purple, but it would be fine to add a red candle as well, to call out romantic love and the expansion you are looking for in that sphere. Amethyst is your friend; take any you may have and put it on your altar or hold it in your hand. You may also lie down for this meditation, and put the stone on your third eye. Do it! Look how groovy you are.

Having lit your candles, incense, what have you, take some oil and draw a star on your third eye. If you have a particular oil that feels good for such a ritual, use it; lavender oil is good, as is any basic oil such as almond or olive. Don't gob it on, go light. Now get to meditating.

Focus on your third eye. Imagine a purple pinwheel spinning there. Maybe a purple bicycle wheel, or one of those twirling firecrackers, spinning electric purple sparks. The motion should be clockwise. You are not asking your third eye for anything, your third eye is *you*, and that connection to the divine is also you. What you are doing is looking for what you already have. You are already an infinite, compassionate Goddexx-like being. You already know how to see beyond the physical, to hop the needle out of its rut and into a whole new groove. You know how to see beauty everywhere, not just where it's obvious or instructed. You know how to live beyond your ego, and you want to connect with others who are working to get behind that numbing trance master.

Repeat this meditation daily, as often as needed, until you feel a bump in your consciousness, until things begin to feel different. And, who knows, you might want to keep it up as a permanent part of your practice, even after you have mastered connecting on a soul level with the people around you. There is always room to ascend.

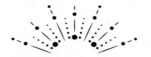

APPENDIX

MODERN MAGIC BOOK LIST/ MY BOOKSHELVES

Being a solo witch, I get most of my information and inspiration from books. I've been devouring spiritual books since I was a teenager, and here are some that really stand out. I'm including some tarot decks and books as well, because a wise tarot deck is a powerful teacher.

TAROT

She Wolfe Tarot, by Devany Amber Wolfe
Thoth Tarot Deck, by Aleister Crowley and Lady Frieda Harris
The Secret Dakini Oracle, by Nik Douglas and Penny Slinger

BOOKS

Jambalaya: The Natural Woman's Book of Personal Charms and Practical Rituals, by Luisah Tiesh
Tarot: Mirror of the Soul, by Gerd Ziegler (for use with *Thoth Tarot*)
The Modern Witch's Spellbook, by Sarah Lyddon Morrison
New Moon Astrology: The Secret of Astrological Timing to Make All Your Dreams Come True, by Jan Spiller
365 Tarot Spreads: Revealing the Magic in Each Day, by Sasha Graham
When Things Fall Apart: Heart Advice for Difficult Times and *The Places That Scare You: A Guide to Fearlessness in Difficult Times,* by Pema Chödrön
Cutting Through Spiritual Materialism, by Chögyam Trungpa
Enchantments: A Modern Witch's Guide to Self-Possession, by Mya Spalter
Wormwood Star: The Magickal Life of Marjorie Cameron, by Spencer Kansa

APPENDIX

The Secret Language of Birthdays and *The Secret Language of Relationships*, by
Gary Goldschneider and Joost Elffers

The Power of Breathwork: Simple Practices to Promote Wellbeing, by Jennifer
Patterson

Seventy-Eight Degrees of Wisdom: A Tarot Journey to Self-Awareness and *A Walk Through
the Forest of Souls: A Tarot Journey to Spiritual Awakening*, by Rachel Pollack

*Llewellyn's Book of Magical Correspondences: A Comprehensive and Cross-Referenced
Resource for Pagans and Wiccans*, by Sandra Kynes

The Way of the Tarot: The Spiritual Teacher in the Cards, by Alejandro Jodorowsky

Tarot (The Library of Esoterica, Taschen), by Jessica Hundley et al.

Zen Mind, Beginner's Mind: Informal Talks on Meditation and Practice and *Not
Always So: Practicing the True Spirit of Zen*, by Shunryu Suzuki

Lovingkindness: The Revolutionary Art of Happiness, by Sharon Salzberg

*Hexing the Patriarchy: 26 Potions, Spells and Magical Elixirs to Embolden the
Resistance* and *We Were Witches*, by Ariel Gore

The Holographic Universe, by Michael Talbot

African Goddess Initiation: Sacred Rituals for Self-Love, Prosperity, and Joy, by
Abiola Abrams

Encyclopedia of 5,000 Spells, by Judika Illes

The Witches: Salem, 1692, by Stacy Schiff

The Chakra Bible, by Patricia Mercier

Who Is Wellness For?, by Fariha Róisín

In Sensorium: Notes for My People, by Tanaïs

The Only Astrology Book You'll Ever Need, by Joanna Martine Woolfolk

The Pocket Book of Stones: Who They Are and What They Teach, by Robert Simmons

You Were Born for This: Astrology for Radical Self-Acceptance, by Chani Nicholas

Courage to Change: One Day at a Time in Al-Anon

Initiated: Memoir of a Witch, by Amanda Yates Garcia

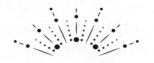

ACKNOWLEDGMENTS

I would like to thank Anna Paustenbach and Chantal Tom for being the most excellent editorial team, and for the sweet energy they brought to this book. Thanks to Rakesh Satyal for jumping in, to Ryan Amato, and to the team at HarperOne. It's been a joy working with you! To Alison Lewis, whose support and humor and smarts I am grateful for on the regular. To Vera Blossom, whose presence in my life is a radical gift. For everyone who made the *Your Magic* podcast happen: Benjamin Cooley, Molly Elizalde, Tony Gannon, Kirsten Osei-Bonsu, Raven Yamamoto, Kristine Mar, and Veronica Agard. Thank you to friends who are always up for a mystical adventure: Peter, Deez, Tara, Nicole, Clement, Beth, Brooke, Kirk, Darren, Clint, Seamus, and Ali. Thank you to practitioners whose work has informed and influenced my own: Chani Nicholas, Marcella Kroll, Sarah Potter, Rhiannon Morsch, Larry Arrington, Lisa Stardust, Edgar Fabián Frias, Mya Spalter, Ariel Gore, Terra Horton, Janae Archuleta, Jessica Hundley, Eliza Swann, and Anna Marie Wood. I'd also like to thank my son, Atticus, for giving me space to work on this book when needed, and my mom, Terri, for helping with that. Some of this work was created at the glorious New Roots Residency; thank you for nurturing queer writers! Final thanks to my beloved incubus, TJ Payne.